DENISE MESSENGER

GOT
CANCER?
NOW
WHAT?

A LAYPERSON'S GUIDE FOR THE NEWLY DIAGNOSED

D1160761

Knowledgeworks Publishing, Costa Mesa, California

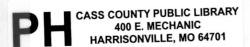

Library of Congress Cataloging-In-Publication Data
Messenger, Denise, 2012
Got Cancer? Now What? A Layperson's Guide for the Newly Diagnosed—1st ed.
Includes bibliographical references and index
1.Cancer—Patients   2. Cancer—Treatment
3.Cancer—Patients—Care—and book, manual,etc.
4. Cancer—Treatment—Decision making

ISBN 978-0-9846820-0-3

ISBN 978-0-9846820-1-0

2011943063

First Edition

Disclaimer

To Stan and Blaine. The two forces behind all my dreams whose loving support made them all come true.

Acknowledgements

To my son Blaine for his constant encouragement, uncanny wisdom in his youth, unquestionable love, devotion and always being by my side. To my sister Melanie for her faith in me, comforting smile and pushing me beyond my limits to accomplish what seemed the impossible. To Helen, my anchor who has held me together through the worst of times and shared the joy in the best of times. To Roberta, for her steady and thoughtful consultations, relentless determination and unwavering faith that a cure was out in the universe waiting for me. To Maureen, who is the wind beneath my sails and my steady compass.

To Dr. Leigh Erin Connealy, Dr. Warren Fong, Dr. Robert Nagourney, John Lu and Bob Xu. All contributed to the writing of this book and were, and continue to be, my "super team" who work tirelessly for their patients, possess the passion, patience and expertise to answer the calling of our ultimate goal—sustain and save lives! To all of you I am eternally grateful.

Contents

Chapter 1
Introduction to Cancer

As I am putting the final changes on this book, I have come to realize what a momentous time this is. It has been well over two years of writing. I often wondered during this process if I would be able to see it through to the finish. There were days of feeling unwell but pushing forward with writing anyway. However, for the most part, the writing was so easy and the research so engrossing that time just flew by.

The most challenging part of writing this was opening up my very guarded and private life to readers I do not know and who do not know me. Readers, by the conclusion of this book, will know the role cancer played in my life and how it translated into benefiting others. I am providing reliable and worthwhile information to the newly diagnosed and others who have experienced similar struggles. I wrote this guide from the heart for every cancer patient and for all people who touch their everyday lives.

This is a layperson's guide, written from a cancer survivor's point of view. You will learn what cancer is and the steps involved in obtaining cancer treatment for you or a loved one. There also is a wealth of information on measures to take for basic survival, including how to maintain everyday activities and continue to thrive. My priority is to provide information for achieving success in treatment and increasing your odds of survival. I want this to be an easy and practical read—a reference to carry with you. I do not want to overwhelm you as a reader or write a voluminous book.

With no formal medical training or scientific background, it has been an exploration in my own diagnosis and in writing this book. Learning medical terminology, scientific verbiage, deciphering clinical studies, tests and medical journals has been challenging. Those very challenges, though, resulted in uncovering meaningful pieces of information. It also was nice to have had the advantage of working for a primary care medical physician for over two years. I am privileged to have met physicians from all over the United States and to have learned about new treatments that were available for cancer.

My cancers were first diagnosed in 2004, and I started treatment soon after. It took six years of systematic research to find treatment protocols to rid me of both types of cancer. It was an uneasy journey, which consisted of a precarious balance between self-experimentation with various methods of treatment and the guidance and advice of many physicians and practitioners. I did not go this alone and it was not "luck" that saved me.

Physicians provide the scientific, technical and medical information regarding a diagnosis. Laboratories provide test results that are often difficult to understand unless you are a scientist, physician or surgeon. At time of diagnosis, vital information is usually communicated quickly or not in great detail. It is often easy to be confused, full of unanswered questions and wondering, "Did I hear them right?" You could also be in shock and feeling fear and panic. The "fear" and "panic" part—that was certainly me!

In talking with cancer patients, one common complaint I hear repeatedly is how devastating it is to get a cancer diagnosis. As alluded to earlier, this is especially true if one is unfortunate enough to get a physician with a poor bedside manner. It can be hard to understand why such a life-changing diagnosis some-times is delivered in such an unfeeling or uncaring way. There could be several reasons for this. One could be that it is normal behavior to rush through appointments as mandated by insur-ance carriers. Another could be that physicians are trying to keep on schedule with all of their appointments and not keep anyone waiting too long. Sometimes physicians are protecting themselves emotionally. And—another reason? Being human, there are times when we all experience a bad day of events!

In retrospect, I guess there is no good way of telling a patient they have cancer. However, physicians giving this life-changing diagnosis could be more sensitive to the patient's utter shock in hearing the news. Yes, there are legal implications involved in giving a patient less than accurate information, but that is not what I am talking to you about. There is always hope, and the strength of the human spirit we should never disregard. No one can predict how a patient will respond to treatment, so why not look on the bright side.

Compassion can go a long way and you want your diagnosis and treatment plan options delivered in a humane fashion. The day you and your family receive the diagnosis is the day every-one's lives change forever. You now are a member of a new club, which by the way, you never wanted to join.

A cancer diagnosis is not only difficult for the new cancer patient to process, but also for their loved ones and friends. However, being in denial and complacent can cause a new set of problems. Life is not fair. Statistically, 10% of the population never recovers from a traumatic event. It is the other 90% who know how to react and actually do who make it through. The ultimate curse is self-pity. The famous saying, "Make lemonade out of lemons" exists for a reason.

I distinctly remember meeting with my surgeon in her conference room to go over my breast cancer diagnosis. When it was time to leave and I was walking down the hall, my doctor asked in a panic if I intended to return for treatment. It struck me odd at the time and I said that I would. "Why are you asking me that?" I asked. She replied, "Because some patients don't return after diagnosis and do nothing." She told me on occasion a patient would go into denial after diagnosis and delay seeking treatment.

Denial is a normal human reaction, but it has no place here. Life is worth fighting for. You mean everything to your friends and family. There is a famous quote by C. Northcote Parkinson that is especially meaningful in this context. He said "Delay is the deadliest form of denial."

Although everyone struggles with denial to some degree, I was mostly filled with questions. Growing up the oldest child of five siblings, I was always the inquisitive one, asking "Why?" all the time. I now realize it was much to my advantage in saving my life. Therefore, when diagnosed, it was no surprise I would be asking "Why?" It became a game of Clue—which by the way, was my favorite board game as a child. I beat all the adults.

So, "Whodunit?" Was I born with a weakness in my DNA? Or was it from secondhand smoke inhalation in my household with smoking parents? Or the 240z Nissan I drove for over five years in my early twenties? Yes, indeed, I breathed in carcinogenic benzene fumes from a bothersome small gas leak for more years than I would like to admit. Oh! Being young and feeling invincible. Or was it the X-rays I received because of scoliosis at the height of my growth spurt? How about the fifteen disintegrating, very large mercury fillings in my mouth I was sucking on the past 25 years? Or maybe living near a landfill and breathing in methane gas or living close to an airport for eleven years and breathing in emissions from the planes? How would I ever really know? I could try to make an educated guess, but it would just be conjecture.

When experiencing cancer, the toughest part of the journey for me was in understanding the chemistry inside my body. My first question was "Why did this happen to me? Two cancers?" I watched what I ate, exercised and never smoked, overused alcohol or used recreational drugs. This was crazy stuff. What did I do to deserve this? Chronic lymphocytic leukemia (CLL) is more common in older men around age 70 than in women. And breast cancer, that was also surprising. Great, I thought—just won the lottery!

For those of you without tangible symptoms or tumors visible or felt by touch, such as in lung cancer, a diagnosis can seem unbelievable. One may outwardly look healthy so it absolutely makes no sense at all. In life, clear explanations for what happens to us are at times hard to find. With cancer, we do have some answers. They present themselves as ones we never thought of before.

So, being me, I had extensive tests to see what was going on in my body. It is amazing what our bodies can deal with and how we have the uncanny ability to adjust over time to the "new normal" no matter how badly we might feel.

I had my hormones checked—estrogen levels off the charts! I had a test to see what my digestive tract was doing—had leaky gut syndrome! Nothing digested well! What else? My thyroid levels were low, and so was Vitamin D. Guess what else was off the charts: white blood cell (WBC) counts and estrogen. Oh, and my progesterone counts were low.

Gee—a strange picture of poor health was emerging. "How could my health reportedly be so bad?" I did not consider myself old enough for all of these health issues. My doctor said, "Your warranty is up!" Now, it would be preventative maintenance along with a major tune-up. What happened? I exercised like crazy and believed I ate well. Actually, though, my nutritionist found that I was not eating as well as I thought. I went through lots of tests and found vitamin and mineral deficiencies. Could the picture get any clearer?

When we started taking a hard look inside my magical body of "Oz," it was eye opening! I needed a major overhaul. My immune system, digestive tract and bone marrow were under attack and I wanted to find out why. Nothing would change until I decided to seek treatment and probably would mean developing an entirely new lifestyle.

At the time of my diagnosis, it would have been very helpful to find a layperson's guide with explanations and suggestions on the steps to take to locate and receive the maximum benefit from physicians, tests and available treatments. Instead, I went on a journey for information by talking to and reading about cancer survivors, as well as talking to physicians, scientists and authors for suggestions on what to do.

This was a time when encouragement and hope were high on my list. I really felt that my life was at stake and the treatment protocol I signed up for was really going to matter. When I had to make a decision on which way to go in treatment, I felt there was a 50/50 chance of being right or wrong and my life depended upon it.

To complicate things, I had vivid images in my head of getting quite sick from treatments, looking and perhaps being close to death's door and possibly losing the will to live. Perhaps since I perceived it to be true, it must be, right?

The other issue for me was the consequences of entering into the medical world of diagnostic testing, probing, consultations and physical exams. Retaining my dignity and modesty was a constant challenge. I recall times of just sobbing during tests, both because of the intrusiveness and out of fear of the results.

Chemotherapy and radiation therapy have come to be synonymous with nausea. I have never coped well with nausea and it has always required me to lie down. It is never a question of toughing it out—I'm down for the count! So, given that realization, a treatment protocol excluding both of those treatment options was high on my wish list.

Another issue is I painfully witnessed two dear friends die from cancer, and their treatment protocols were brutally hard! The mental images and emotional trauma from those experiences will be with me forever.

It was my desire going into treatment to have full knowledge of the disease and the challenges ahead to better equip myself for the physical, mental and emotional journey. What was foremost in my mind was to survive treatment and experience a good quality of life. At all costs, my cherished hair was going to stay on my head! Call it vain or whatever you want; it was just another reason why chemotherapy was not an option if it could take my hair away from me. There had to be another way.

I had specific questions that needed answers. They were:

- Why did this happen to me? What was the cause of my cancer?
- What did the test results tell the physicians?
- How accurate were the tests and the technicians conducting them?
- How experienced were the physicians interpreting the test results, and how good was their judgment?
- What treatment protocols were available?
- What were the downsides to certain treatments?
- How would the treatments benefit me specifically?
- Would I end up better or worse off from certain treatments?
- Whom could I trust?

These questions were important and I was determined to find the answers and receive treatments to wipe out these cancers and spare my life. I spent endless hours on the internet, in libraries and bookstores, reading and buying a multitude of books, research papers, and magazine articles to search for answers. I scheduled office visits with nutrition experts, medical physicians, surgeons, acupuncturists, herbalists, consultants and as mentioned earlier, even worked for a medical physician.

After my diagnoses with cancer, I never suffered from the flu and only had a cold once in seven years. However, my immune system and stamina weakened as the CLL progressed. I was also at high risk for infection. Activities outside of my home were kept to a minimum. This meant no large crowds of people or extended travel. I needed to find an effective treatment soon.

Just in the nick of time, as a Stage IV cancer patient, I agreed to a chemotherapy treatment in which there would be no sickness or loss of hair. Prior to treatment, my oncologist said he was surprised and amazed to find no history of serious infections.

Other than having cancer, I was relatively healthy. It was reassuring to hear that I was in good shape to withstand chemotherapy by several of my physicians. I knew on a completely new level that I could do it, especially because of prior treatments that required many years of good nutrition, supplements, acupuncture, and working on issues that caused stress in my life.

During chemotherapy treatments, I found it to be true that there was no hair loss, nausea or weight loss. Hallelujah! Instead, I gained weight and enjoyed every single solitary meal. However, let me caution you! This is not what others might experience. Age can make a difference and everyone has different chemistry and has treated their bodies differently over time. In treating cancer, many different drugs and therapy protocols produce various side effects. However, treatment without the negative side effects is a great goal for everyone.

One of the most damaging things a person can do during this journey is to worry and let fear become the controlling factor in making decisions. Waiting for test results is incredibly unnerving, but the best thing to do is not jump to conclusions. Our bodies have an innate ability to heal. Getting medical treatment is one thing, but having a positive emotional and mental outlook plays a big role, too.

Stress can be a killer and may actually contribute to the development of cancer. Find the triggers that create stress in your life and eliminate them. Stay calm and keep focused on healing; this is imperative for recovery. One way or the other, you will get through this. If you are in need of a touch, a smile or a kind word, reach out to the people who love you.

Chapter 2
For the Newly Diagnosed

Worldwide, more than 7.5 million people died of cancer and 12 million new cases were diagnosed in 2007 according to the International Cancer Genome Consortium. Unless there is medical progress, the numbers could rise to 17.5 million deaths and 27 million new cases in 2050.

These statistics reflect a troublesome trend relative to cancer. The projections are that one out of every three people in their lifetime will get cancer. What alarmingly high numbers considering we have been raging a war on cancer for almost four decades. Our past president Richard M. Nixon signed The National Cancer Act (P.L. 92–218) (a.k.a. "The War on Cancer") in 1971. This bill appropriated $100 million to launch an intensive campaign to find a cure for cancer, and the United States now spends billions of dollars each year fighting cancer.

Very few of us know what cancer is from a scientific standpoint. We just know that it has the ability to dismantle lives. We read or hear about it on the news. Some loved one, family member, acquaintance or friend ends up with it. It is the dreaded "word" and if it happens to you, it feels like a death threat, something difficult to process.

I thought my body had betrayed me. Because of stories I had heard about cancer victims and from my friends' experiences with cancer, pain, fear and anxiety overwhelmed me. Ridding myself of the feeling of helplessness took some time. It was quite profound to wake up in the morning out of a deep sleep realizing that what I had to deal with was still there. Oh, how nice! It was waiting just for me, the chosen one! It was not a dream. It would not disappear unless forced out of my body and mind. The diagnostic tests and biopsies had confirmed it. I remember thinking about ignoring it. Maybe it would all go away! Maybe the bump or lump was benign and no big deal. It was a good-feeling place for the moment but a very bad-feeling place for my future.

How could one word—cancer—have so much power over me? The ultimate answer was that there really is no power in just a word unless you buy into it! Life always has challenges—this is just one more. The mystery is in what will be uncovered in the following weeks and months after diagnosis. There will be good and bad days throughout the process. The best way to stabilize emotions is to take one day at a time.

When you are diagnosed, you might not question your physicians or therapies and will do precisely what the first trained medical professional you visit says. This may be done out of sheer panic. It is understandable, but the fact is that spending time researching other alternatives can result in significantly different (and potentially better) outcomes.

What if as a patient you decided to be less compliant? Why do you have to go through certain procedures, surgeries, treatments and to what end? Will the treatments prolong your life for a while or cure you? Another question might be whether treatments will possibly aggravate your disease.

We all have different personalities and differ in our ways of dealing with crises. I have observed some people who are warrior-like and take charge of their care experience better outcomes than those who are submissive from the beginning. For people of faith and/or have a strong determination to beat cancer, healing is possible and there are many survivors to prove it. We beat the odds all the time and do phenomenally well. Sometimes the medical establishment has no explanations for those who survive against the odds.

One good quality to have is to trust in your instincts. Once you have thought about all the research, have considered physician opinions, and have made a final decision for treatment, do not over-think the decision. Fully commit to the treatment, be confident with your decision and be at peace with it. You will find out soon enough if it is working.

What is particularly important in this process is to avoid panic. Panic accelerates the disease because it creates additional stress on the body and breaks down tissue. Find a sense of calm before making critical decisions.

I recall a time when one of my oncologists told me to get my affairs in order and immediately report to the hospital due to a fractured spleen. He also wanted to start chemotherapy treatment. This meant that I should prepare my Will and get a Power of Attorney because of the possibility I would likely not survive. It scared the living daylights out of me, but I had the inner strength to reach deep down and assess my circumstances. My intuition advised me differently and I obtained another opinion. I received a different treatment; and am here to share my story!

Many cancer patients report having experienced major stress in their lives six to 18 months prior to the onset of their illness. They confess to pushing themselves beyond their limits in either physical, mental or emotional domains (or a combination of the three). This could be due to a change or loss of a job, a bad marriage, relationship, divorce, death, illness, an accident or feeling you were wronged by someone.

Cancer patients who let bygones be bygones and take personal responsibility for their health are ahead of the game. In examining one's participation in life, look for major life changes or unhappiness. Is there a negative relationship or job dissatisfaction? Have you become an "empty nester" with kids off to college or moved out of the household? Was there a death in the family or broken relationship? Have you neglected a reasonable diet, sleep or exercise? All these things can contribute to poor health and psyche.

Look within your deeper self, find your triggers and do something about them. I am a strong proponent of the "mind-body" connection. Looking for a cure is personal. What goes a long way is your belief in yourself and the people who will be with you through the process of recovery. Stress is a killer and a happy and balanced emotional life is necessary for beating cancer.

Make cancer an inspiring challenge and not a threat. I had gratitude toward everyone helping me and it brought a certain level of happiness. Your thinking is something you have control over. Your mind and spirit are not owned by cancer. Get rid of negative baggage and revamp your life. Decide from the first day of diagnosis to change what is not working in your life, do what you love and keep doing it throughout your treatment.

I have a friend who went shopping after each weekly chemotherapy treatment for breast cancer. Her love for clothes shopping made her happy, so she would treat herself once a week. Do what makes you happy and feels good. Continue living life. It is yours for the taking.

In this journey, get the proper information to make informed decisions. Get in touch with family, friends, support groups, therapists, and religious organizations. Perhaps explore your inner self. Look at ways to improve your home environment for healing. Improve nutrition. Get plenty of sleep for healing and find ways to relax.

Find ways to inspire yourself. When I was going through therapy, I had different experiences depending upon the day. I chose happiness because otherwise I felt it would not find me. For example, on my first day of chemotherapy we had to wait in the office hallway because the physician's staff was still out to lunch. As I waited, I used the iPad my son had given me as a gift. He knew there would be long hours involved in therapy and that the iPad would keep me entertained. He is smart knowing—I would have pestered him for hours on end! I picked an inspirational piece of music from the iPad to stay in the right frame of mind because I was very nervous. So nervous, in fact, I was jiggling around in my shoes and slightly swaying to the music. While listening to the music, I was telling myself how excited I was to be getting chemotherapy because it was going to get me well. I recall that experience now and think I must have been half out of my mind with anxiety!

Not soon after, a man showed up with his wife. He looked at me with contempt, shook his head, looked down at the floor and shuddered. I could feel his pain. A few minutes later, I heard his pain. He asked me how I could be dancing and appear to be so happy. I just smiled at him. Even though I was anxious, I just looked happy! It was easy to see that he was living his worst nightmare. His wife explained he was not eating and was feeling sick because of chemotherapy and was having a bad week. He had difficulty getting out of bed to come to the doctor's office. He was dehydrated and coming in for fluids. As it turns out, I continued to see him from week to week and his health improved. His face lit up one day when I offered him an organic drink full of nutrients, which I drank regularly. He said it tasted good and drank the entire bottle, so his wife ordered them for him with the doctor's approval. She was thrilled to see he found something that appealed to him and he was getting some good nutrition. Bringing some light into his life that day and showing him some compassion brought me joy!

I experienced many different emotions throughout my experience, such as forgiveness, self-love, compassion and appreciation for life. Faith, family, and friends were at the top of my support tree. Find yours, too.

Chapter 3
First Steps

Never in your life will you have so many questions with so little time to answer them before needing to take action. Medical professionals will make determinations about your disease based on physical examinations, blood tests, urinalyses, biopsies, bone scans, positron emission tomography (PET) scans, magnetic resonance imaging (MRIs), X-rays and pathology reports. Depending upon the cancer diagnosis and prognosis, you may have the luxury of waiting and researching. However, a physician may tell you "time is of the essence" and treatment must commence immediately, which could mean within days or weeks.

If you have a full-time job, there is little free time to do the many hours of research necessary, let alone go to all the doctor's and diagnostic appointments. The stress of seeing medical professionals, having conversations with family members and friends and continuing to work will sometimes seem to be more than you can handle.

When the going gets tough, take a break and do something that makes you laugh. Laughter can be healing because it increases killer T-cell activity in the body, which boosts the immune system.' Watch a funny movie, go see a comedy or read a good book. Do anything to take your mind away from cancer.

When I received the breast cancer diagnosis in 2004, I knew I had a challenging disease. Little did I know that later on after lymph node dissection, a diagnosis of CLL also was all mine! My oncologist diagnosed CLL prior to scheduled surgery because my WBC counts were high (19,000) even though I felt fine. Sometimes high WBC counts in this range are associated with the flu.

When I had a lumpectomy, it was a relief to find that breast cancer was not in my lymph nodes. However, CLL was. The memory of this life-changing event is always with me. When I woke up from surgery and was in recovery, my surgeon told me I had Lymphoma and needed chemotherapy or I could die. She said the breast cancer was not as big of an issue. My family in the waiting room also heard the same thing and became frightened.

I became hysterical once I got home and was in bed yelling, "I don't want to die!" When the anesthesia wore off and I could think clearly, I told my family everything was under control. I recalled my previous conversation with my oncologist that the CLL diagnosis was a slow growing form and needed no treatment at the time. Some people lived into old age with it.

I give this example to point out that doing your homework (research and seeing specialists) and communicating back to your team of physicians is so important for answering questions later. If I had communicated the suspected CLL diagnosis to my surgeon earlier, the experience would never have taken place. My surgeon was acting in my best interest at the time.

CLL is not a common cancer and effective treatment options were limited to ongoing clinical trials in 2001. Money for CLL research was not substantial in comparison to other types of cancer research. Patient outcomes with this disease were not good in my eyes. I needed to stay alive and bide my time until something new came along.

The accepted protocol at the time of my diagnosis was to "watch and wait" before starting treatment. It remains the same to this day. Based on my extensive blood and genetic testing, the CLL appeared to be indolent (slow growing), but no one could guarantee it would stay that way. I had two types of cancer and understood why everyone was pushing me to do something about the breast cancer first. I longed to do the right thing and often wondered—what and—when? My biggest challenge was sorting through what everyone had to say, determining the accuracy of the information, finding my own truth and either accepting or not accepting advice before taking action.

I have to say making the right decision about treatments can be a long and tedious process. I literally would see a physician one day and be convinced their protocol was the way to go and then wake up the next morning with my gut yelling "Hell, no!" Listen to your inner self. It never misled me.

Having the luxury of time to research the options available in my situation was possible after my biopsy. On a scale of one to ten (with ten being the most aggressive form), my breast tumor was a two. I always try to find the positive in everything, so two was something positive to work with. The less aggressive the tumor, the better off I hoped I would be.

Making the decision in 2004 to treat my breast cancer surgically via lumpectomy without chemotherapy or radiation was an agonizing decision. I made this decision because there was no lymph node involvement, even though my physicians advised against it. Based on the literature at the time, and considering my particular situation, I was not convinced that harsh chemotherapy would be beneficial for treating my breast cancer. I believed surgery alone would take care of it and that chemotherapy and radiation would have weakened my immune system further, possibly aggravating the CLL. Through my research, I also found a small possibility of heart muscle or lung damage after radiation to the left breast, with life-threatening consequences later down the road, so I decided to opt out.[2,3] Due to this decision and the use of alternative measures and different therapies, I have not had a reoccurrence of breast cancer and am cured.

Once I decided that surgery was the way to go, I needed to determine whether my surgeon could clear the margins of the tumor during my lumpectomy. Clearing the margins means that the tumor needs to be extracted in such a way that the tissue around the tumor site is free of cancerous cells. Depending on the location of the tumor, this can be tricky in the first surgery. Finding a good surgeon is very important!

The next order of business, after much research, was to bring my body back to a healthy state. This would take a great deal of work, especially because of the lack of research examining the breakdown of the immune system in cancer. Decades of research has vacillated between exploring whether a virus causes cancer or whether it is largely a genetic mutation.[4] These research questions continue to lead to many unanswered questions. One thing known is that environmental components are a factor in causing a breakdown in immune function causing cancer.

Regardless of what I found during my research, cancer was a fact in my life. I decided to work on bringing my immune system up to a healthier level, increase my killer T-cell production to help kill the cancer cells and strengthen my immune function, detoxify any possible contaminant exposures I may have had and add in some good nutrition.

I needed to locate physicians experienced in these areas to help me. This was challenging. It turned into an exercise of Who? What? Where? My view was that even with all the research I had done, trying unproven methods or using certain herbs, supplements or vitamins unsupervised could be detrimental to my recovery. I needed to surround myself with people who had experience—lots and lots of people. The process was tough, time consuming, expensive, and emotionally painful. My entire life, at work and home, turned upside down. However, looking back on all of this now, I was decisive, made brave decisions and was very successful in overcoming breast cancer and, ultimately, CLL.

The Emotional Factor

I have chosen to discuss the emotional factor in the battle with cancer because we often only think of the physical aspects of the fight. One challenge I never anticipated right after diagnosis was how people would react to the news. I experienced an emotional rollercoaster for which I wasn't prepared. Very close family members disagreed with what I wanted to do. Others did not give me any advice at all, foregoing all responsibility. Who could really blame them? No one wanted to shoulder responsibility for a poor outcome. Others exclaimed, "It is much too difficult to make a critical life-saving decision for you with the current information at hand, and I am not a doctor!" I agreed and understood. No one should carry the heavy burden except me, along with my physicians. In moments of weakness, though, I hoped someone else would.

The most you can hope for is that people will be supportive of whatever you choose. I had some family and friends I thought would support me emotionally through the horrific experience completely disappear. I never heard from them again. Some popped up after it was all over and I was just fine. Some were right by my side the entire time, whereas others took a "sideline" approach by checking in every couple of months. I have a large network of family and friends so I considered myself quite fortunate in receiving plenty of love, kindness and support.

People who care about you want to communicate their emotions and thoughts, but sometimes keep quiet out of fear of saying or doing the wrong thing. I found some to be plain scared of the entire situation, so much so they scared themselves away. They had very little knowledge of how cancer works and had no interest in learning. I had what they never wanted to have or even think about it. For a year or more, some of my old friends who knew about my cancer didn't call me out of fear I had died!

It was a painful time both physically and emotionally. Some people expressed a true sadness, almost pity. I am much too proud for that, so there were friends and other people in my life I never told. It just was not worth it. Besides, sometimes it was a well needed escape to walk around knowing my neighbors, some friends and business acquaintances were void of the truth.

In a way, writing this guide was rather therapeutic even though thinking about my experience still brings tears to my eyes. The tears are for people to whom I am eternally grateful, and who I love and respect with everything in me. My family, along with old and new friends were with me every step along the way. They are the angels of this world! Aside from relying on your own, joining a support group can be beneficial. Cancer blogs and web sites on the internet are also popular.

People have complex emotions along with busy and hectic lives. They react and help the best way they know how at the time of your illness. Forgiveness is something you will learn a lot about in the months and years to come, and compassion is something you will experience time-and-time again. However, people who can step outside their own pain long enough to help you with yours truly know how to love. Find them!

If you talk to cancer survivors, almost all have a renewed outlook on life. When I meet a fellow cancer survivor for the first time, there is an immediate bond. Cancer survivors have a renewed spirit. Some who were never religious or spiritual become so. People who had a strong belief system and were of faith had their prayers answered. Others are just glad to be here for whatever reasons. They overcame an unimaginable silent enemy from within. Some have unstoppable perseverance and feelings of value and self-worth. Some cancer survivors go forward in life taking nothing for granted. Sometimes survival is so random. Survivors may work toward accomplishing long sought-after goals (bucket lists) and developing new goals in life.

Families change forever—for the good, the bad and the ugly. It takes inner strength to survive cancer and recognized through many people's eyes as being one of the "lucky" ones. For me, I have chosen to head in an entirely new direction in life-to help others and live for a greater purpose. I cherish every new day and appreciate the small things. As a cancer survivor I have received the grand prize—life! I will never take it for granted.

The choice of which treatment to pursue is critical for positive outcomes. For every type of cancer, there are many treatment options available in the United States and all over the world. I found the trick to treatment protocols is to know when to fold if the treatment appears to be doing more harm than good. Let it go and move on to the next. If you are the type of person who always has to finish projects, no matter what—rethink that notion! Taking risks is part of the process. If you find it difficult to take risks, now is the time to change! If you consider yourself shy—become a bulldog! It is for your own good. Time is of the essence. Research, analyze your options and always have a back-up plan. Make decisions based on what fits your situation and never give up because there is an answer to everything. You may not be satisfied with the answers you get so find others!

Hospitalization

If you, a family member or friend is hospitalized it is important for someone to be in the hospital room at all times as an advocate. Hospitals at times are understaffed due to budget restraints and cutbacks. Your immediate needs are no more important than the needs of other patients. If there is a serious drug reaction, fall out of bed or other life-threatening event, the staff may not be immediately available because they are busy with other patients at the same time. Your advocate can also assist in the avoidance of infection, drug errors and surgical mistakes.

In a study published in November of 2010 by the United States Office of Inspector General for the Department of Health and Human Services, findings concluded that an estimated 13.5% of hospitalized Medicare patients (one out of every seven) were harmed requiring additional medical intervention during their hospitalizations. Hospital infections contributed to the problem, but other events were more common. Approximately 180,000 patients per year were harmed due to medications, excessive bleeding, intravenous fluid overload, and surgery. Patients experienced either a temporary setback or even death during their hospitalization. The most serious events, such as operating on the wrong patient, amounted to less than 1% of such errors.[5] In 2011, an estimated 187,000 deaths in hospitals were due to adverse medical events and medical interventions separate from the underlying medical condition.[6]

As a patient or advocate, ask questions and demand answers in order to reduce errors. Make sure all physicians and medical staff wash their hands before your examinations or treatments. This helps to lower the possibility of infection which you do not want. When a medication is prescribed for you, find out why and determine the potential side effects. Check for multiple medication interactions. Prior to surgery, make sure you consult with your physician to review the procedure. After surgery, have devices no longer needed removed as soon as possible to cut down on the risk of infection.

Medical Insurance

Medical insurance in the United States has become cumbersome, expensive and for some unobtainable. Medical insurance companies and government run programs complicate our lives with policies, procedures and regulations. It has become increasingly difficult to treat patients in a cost-effective manner and at the same time devote ample time to patient-doctor interactions. Malpractice lawsuits also drive up the cost of care. Physicians perform more and more tests to avoid the potential legal complications of not diagnosing and treating patients properly.

In 2003, physicians' estimated annual liability premiums in the United States reached $26 billion.[7] This amounted to a 2,000% increase since 1975. The average malpractice lawsuit awards were $4.7 million.[8] Physician offices have to add insurance premium costs into their operational expenses, and hospitals pay these premiums for the physicians on their payroll. When considering the small profit margins of hospitals, which as reported in September of 2009 was about 4% for all hospital classes with teaching hospitals at around 6%, there is little room for staying afloat financially.[9]

In 2011, some physicians were closing their private practices due to lower reimbursement rates and continued financial stress. They joined large physician groups. Some of these groups tend to work regular 9 to 5 hours, which could have disastrous consequences due to not being available in cases of emergencies after hours. Instead, in some instances a patient is rushed to an emergency care facility unfamiliar with the patient's health history. We are also continually losing gifted, dedicated and seasoned groups of physicians who are retiring or changing professions. We will see how this plays out in terms of patient care in the years to come.

There are several factors contributing to the closing of hospitals, including the high number of unpaid and unreimbursed emergency room visits by the uninsured, as well as Medicare cuts and lower reimbursement rates. Emergency services are in crisis in certain cities in the United States. Emergency rooms are crowded and patients with or without insurance are often sent to other facilities after initial emergency treatment is completed or are sent home too early. Patients at times could also be transported to other facilities due to insurance issues.

The average emergency room waiting time in most cities is six hours. Our high standards of care undoubtedly suffer at times due to the lack of sufficient time, budget restraints, rules, regulations, and reimbursement rates.

Physicians annually receive lower payments and reimbursement rates for their services from government programs and certain carriers, including some medications. There are large workloads in some areas of the United States and not enough available hospital beds for treatment and admissions. Insurance companies are always looking for ways to cut costs and improve their profit margins. They run like big corporations and report to shareholders. This can result in denial of claims or changes in recommended treatments, which can slow patient recovery. In fact, patients who appeal denials directly to the insurer win 39-59% of the time, depending on the state (only four states collect relevant data) according to a recent report from the Government Accountability Office (GAO).[10]

Patients these days are in the crossfire. It is difficult when patients have to go through medical assessment for treatment, yet are alone in fighting for the best care available with the current financial limitations, regulations and red tape.

Some insurance carriers, facilities and physicians do excellent work in caring for patients. Find them. This could be one of your greatest challenges.

Practitioners have heavy patient loads (sometimes as many as 80-90 patients per day, which can be exhausting). The troubling question is: How can a complicated patient's case be properly assessed in 15 minutes or less? It takes five minutes or more to review a patient's chart!

Years ago, our society believed that cancer was a top priority in terms of treatment with no cost spared. Today, insurance companies and the Centers for Medicare and Medicaid Services are looking to cost containment by grouping patients with specific cancers into standardized treatment protocols and nothing more. This is a troubling trend for patients denied life-saving cancer drugs. Such drugs might be capable of curing them, but because of new rules patients could lose their lives instead.

Insurance companies and the government are not concerned with the operating costs needed to keep physicians' offices open and running. The insurance industry and the government have their budgets and bottom lines to protect. Today, this translates into patients receiving reduced quality of care, rationing of services and the denial of more expensive treatments that could save lives.

We are seeing excellent and dedicated physicians turning away patients because they cannot afford to treat them. The noble profession of doctoring is drowning in paperwork and financially struggling to survive. If this persists, as previously mentioned, fewer physicians will be around to treat us. Medical students will have no incentive to spend up to $400,000 in education to become physicians knowing that they will join a group of physicians owned by a large corporation to make an above average income. Why is this bad? Some physicians lose their authority and autonomy to make individualized patient treatment decisions. For instance, these new physicians could receive quotas on how many operations they can conduct monthly or the alternative measures they must satisfy first, delaying surgery for months. This is rationed care.

Be Prepared for Office Visits

Even though there are many wonderful outcomes for cancer patients at this time, things do slip through the cracks. It is very important to take responsibility during the process of cancer treatment because of the possibility of misdiagnosis, harmful treatment protocols and mistakes. When multiple drugs are prescribed with no account of how they interact with one another; this can kill! Patients who are involved in their care have the power to reduce error rates for better outcomes. Track and double-check every medication, test and procedure. It makes good sense to help an understaffed and overworked nursing and hospital staff.

Taking all of this into consideration, the most important thing to remember is that *one size does not fit all.* As a patient, you have to be your own advocate. We are all individuals, and we need individualized medicine.

It is important to follow-up on every test result and every appointment. Get copies of all tests, including disks of your scans. Depending on what specialist you see, disks are crucial and can expedite the diagnostic process. Some physicians are experts at reviewing scans and may immediately see something missed by others.

So, are you thinking that this is going to be a lot of work? There are very clear reasons why it is worth the effort. Physicians do not have limitless memories. We ask them to be detectives and expect them to know everything about us. None will profess to be mind readers and are usually pressed for time. Providing this information will free up more time for your questions.

Now, for the homework! Bring all your medical records. They should be concise, clear and in chronological order. Make a spreadsheet tracking your blood work. If you have a blood-related cancer, such records are particularly important in tracking your disease. You can obtain a spreadsheet template. by downloading it from www.gotcancernowwhat.com. Put the spreadsheet in a notebook with a historical outline. Include separately marked sections as shown on next page.

• Medications/Supplements
• Radiology results
• Labs
• Hospital admissions/discharge summaries
• Pathology reports
• Notes

Before arriving for a doctor visit, schedule a friend or family member to accompany you for the first consultation. It is an important visit and having a second set of ears is useful in remembering the conversation. If you own a tape recorder, bring it along and ask permission to use it.

The main goal of your first appointment is to understand your disease and explore treatment possibilities. Bring a list of questions. Prioritize your list in case your appointment time is limited. Ten questions is not inappropriate. Bring one copy for the physician to read and one to take notes. In stressful office visits, it is difficult to remember the questions and answers.

It is okay to question treatment protocols and tests with your physician. If you have agreed to a test, know its name and what it is so you can be sure to request (and ultimately receive) the right test when you go to the appointment. If you have any allergies to medications, be sure to let them know.

If you have an uncommon type of cancer, seek out oncologists who are subspecialists—physicians who have devoted their professional lives to your specific type of cancer. Cancer centers and universities are a good place to look. They are much more inclined to be aware of or involved with the latest treatment protocols. You can get a good idea of their level of expertise by the research or clinical studies they discuss or direct you to the year of published research. Specialists will give you general examples of patients they have treated over the years with your type of cancer and what the outcomes were. Some physicians will give you the opportunity to talk with their staff if you have concerns.

It is up to you to assess whether the recommended treatments will be beneficial. Do as much research as possible before consenting to them. I quickly found out that not every physician agreed with the suggested treatment protocols of others. Physicians differ in the programs they administer. These conflicts often left me wondering what to do. It truly can be a balancing act.

All cancers have gene mutations and this is where treatment can get complicated." Once tests reveal what they are and you have researched everything on your particular cancer in question, it never hurts to find an outside cancer consultant to help make sense of it all. Consultants are a neutral third party that receives a fee to review your treatment options. They have backgrounds as chiefs or heads of oncology departments and are typically associated with hospitals, research universities or in private practice. Choose someone with a great deal of experience treating your specific cancer.

Please consider waiting to start treatment until you seek at least three opinions from physicians. The very first physician may recommended the correct therapy, but be sure. This is your life!

If money is an issue in paying for a consultation, borrow it. This is how strongly I believe in the value of consultations. Remember, cancer treatment is a big business and you will be welcomed as a customer everywhere you go to seek treatment. Often physicians will advise you that his or her drugs or treatments are the answer. Maybe yes, maybe no!

According to government officials, the cost of treating cancer in the United States will rise 27% to at least $158 billion by 2020 assuming costs and survival rates remain stable.[12]

Chapter 4
Visiting the Doctor

A doctor visit is a very time-consuming and expensive proposition. There is the loss of work and driving time, the office reception and patient room waits. If you prepare the information mentioned in the previous chapter prior to your visit, it will help maximize the little time you have with the physician. Prior to your doctor visit, call ahead and have forms mailed to your home or download them from their web sites. This will enable you to prepare them ahead of time, reducing your time filling out paperwork in the waiting room.

Keep these points in mind: Once you are in front of the doctor, be concise about your situation. Discuss when your problem started and what your symptoms have been. Tell them whether symptoms have improved or worsened. Explain what treatments you have undergone and whether they have improved your situation or made it worse. Also, be as specific as you can when describing your history.

Bring copies of all your tests. This includes CT scans, MRIs, PET scans, and blood labs. Obtain them from the doctor's offices that ordered them, or get copies from the radiology center on a CD. Always keep a copy for yourself for future visits with other physicians.

Ask the doctor whether there are any other tests recommended for your disease to help in diagnosis or staging. If they recommend a diagnostic test and you are aware of perhaps a better or less invasive test you would like to try, ask them.

Have a written list of no more than ten questions you want answered by your doctor. Hand him/her the questions so you both have copies. Doctors tend to be in a hurry and you need to ask questions quickly and write down the answers for later reference.

Questionnaire for First Doctor Appointment

1. How will you go about confirming my diagnosis? (Not as easy as it sounds!)

2. Biopsy. Do I need one and if so why?

3.   Does a biopsy involve surgery and what are the procedures involved? How long does it take to receive the biopsy result?

4. What other tests do you recommend and why?

5. Will you support the use of complementary supplements, etc. during treatment?

6. How long will it take for a diagnosis?

7. Do you confer with other physicians for treatment protocols?

8. How do you keep up-to-date on new treatments?

9. Are you opposed to reviewing other treatment options recommended to me by other physicians?

10. Will you administer someone else's recommended treatment plan?

Questionnaire Once Diagnosis Confirmed From Tests

1. What are your findings from my test results?

2. What is my prognosis and my chances of a cure?

3. Do you have a treatment plan and for how long?

4. How often will you draw blood and where?

5. How often will tests such as MRI's, CT scans, X-rays, etc. be run during my treatment plan? Are you flexible in the timing of these tests?

6. Is chemotherapy or radiation involved? Is there anything else we could do instead?

7. What are the treatments, drugs and dosages? For how long?

8. How likely will these drugs work on my cancer considering your experience treating other patients with the same prognosis?

9. Do you administer chemotherapy in your office? Do you have a chair for a family member to sit with me during chemotherapy?

10. What challenges am I facing fighting this disease and what will they be? How can we lessen them? Can I still work or go to school?

Chapter 5
Selecting Doctors

Selecting doctors will be the most important challenge in dealing with cancer. The team of experts you put together will include the individuals who walk you through the process. They negate life-threatening side effects and work hard to save your life.

If you own medical insurance, you most likely already have a primary care physician. If you have a HMO, you see physicians within the referral network open to new patients. If you have a PPO, you pick the physician you want (which is a big advantage) and if they are within the insurer's referral network, the costs are less. A PPO also gives you the option to seek multiple opinions from various physicians and specialists. You may choose to visit many physicians outside your network, but reimbursement will be less. The important thing is to be comfortable with your choices and confident you will receive the best care possible.

Research from Harvard Medical School strongly suggests that the length of time a physician has been in practice does not necessarily correlate with the quality of medical care. Instead, seek out physicians trained in treating your specific illness or medical condition and investigate peer and patient reviews.

Some physicians who have practiced medicine for many years may have only treated a small number of patients with your specific cancer. Conversely, newer physicians who have joined practices under the wing of older physicians or who work in cancer center or university settings may have access to the treatment protocols of thousands of patients with the same cancer as you.

Cancer is a whole body, systemic issue, so you will need to find a team of physicians and practitioners that will address the different aspects of getting you well. You might want to locate a physician experienced in conducting or interpreting tests designed to assess your overall health and possible nutritional deficiencies. Every cancer patient has them. Ask whether your attending physician is open to additional blood and urine tests outside of the standard complete blood count (CBC) work to determine your mineral and vitamin levels, along with amino acid and hormone levels. For example, knowing whether there is a deficiency in vitamin D is very important because of its role in immune function. Studies today show evidence of people being on the low side of acceptable ranges. When fighting cancer, high levels are more beneficial.[13]

These days, there is a trend toward physicians encouraging patients to take supplements, but most physicians lack the knowledge or time to counsel patients. Counseling patients in supplements is an acquired skill that physicians must seek out. They have to set aside time outside of work hours to educate themselves through reading and attending conferences or seminars.

Here are some suggestions for helping you find a physician experienced in treating your specific illness: Devise a list of referrals. Your physician may refer you to other physicians in your area. You can also do an internet search of physicians in your area. Once you have the list, look up physicians at the web site www.ama-assn.org, which will give you links to the American Medical Association (AMA) medical boards in your state. You can find out whether physicians have a history of lawsuits or complaints filed against them. It never hurts to know.

Most practicing physicians have hospital privileges. Search the hospitals with which they are associated for their information. Hospital web sites usually show their credentials and years of practice and specialty. If there is an emergency during your treatment, you want to have a physician who has admitting privileges at the hospital with which they are associated.

If the Joint Commission on Accreditation of Healthcare Organizations (JCAHO) accredits a hospital, it is a plus. They are an independent, not-for-profit organization accrediting more than 15,000 health care organizations and programs in the United States. Hospitals that receive accreditation status must undergo rigorous inspections and meet specific standards of performance affecting the quality and safety of patient care. It is advisable to search on the internet for an accredited hospital at www.jointcommission.org.

Once you have looked up this information and are satisfied with the results, start calling physician's offices. Find out whom to talk to about your specific medical condition in terms of how many patients the physician treats during the course of a year. Also, inquire about how many cases like yours they have treated successfully in his or her career. You should be able to start narrowing it down to who can treat you best.

If you want to know how progressive and current a physician is, search for any published articles authored by him or her. There also are many medical journals, newsletters, books and organizations you can search online. Two good sources are www.worldcat.org and www.pubmed.com.

Research whether a physician or consultant you are considering also has a joint faculty appointment at a medical school. If so, they may have more contact with leading medical experts and scientists with up-to-date information on the latest advances in research and treatments than community-based physicians without an affiliation with a medical school.

Look into cancer organizations listed on the internet specializing in your specific cancer. You can find a wealth of information.

Chapter 6
Finding an Oncologist

Oncologists can be very different in their experience levels of treating your type of cancer. Their personalities vary and how they manage their offices. This is a big decision and is going to be the most important physician you hire. You want a correct diagnosis, staging, and treatment, and it can take time to get it all. Two vital attributes that set oncologists apart is whether they have creativity and/or good judgment. Oncologists must also gain your trust in order to have a productive doctor/patient relationship.

I had the pleasure of interviewing a leading oncologist, Dr. Warren Fong, located in Newport Beach, California. He is also a hematologist and internist practicing for 17 years. Dr. Fong is a Fellow in the American College of Physicians (F.A.C.P.). This is a prestigious organization for physicians who practice internal medicine. He was my oncologist and he saved my life. You cannot get any better than that! The information gleaned from him for this guide is invaluable.

Oncologists function as primary care physicians in managing the complex issues associated with cancer. This involves coordinating a diverse collection of medical services that must work together in harmony. This requires oncology skills as well as superior management abilities.

Oncologists set themselves apart by their subspecialties, or the types of cancer they treat. Some are generalists who treat all cancers, whereas others dedicate their lives to one specific cancer and are found working in university medical research centers or in private cancer centers. These specialists see patients in their offices, but patients often have the option of taking their prescribed treatment protocol to an oncologist closer to home.

Oncologists at times collaborate with one another regarding new research and drug therapies. They also enlist the opinions of scientists and PhDs in university research departments for advice on specific cases.

When it comes to what you expect an oncologist to know, keep in mind it is impossible for them to keep up on every new drug, technology and study published. However, what can set them apart is in the creative way they apply new information in their practice. Never be afraid to bring to their attention information you uncovered on your own. It could be extremely valuable. Most want you to ask their opinion about what you have found.

Oncologists and their offices all operate differently. Some oncologists administer chemotherapy in their offices. Such offices have their own administrative staff and registered nurses (RNs), keeping infection rates and mistakes to a minimum. They get to know their patients by name and have their complete medical charts. Medication combinations are prepared in their offices. If drug interactions or illnesses occur your physician can address them immediately, as he or she is in the office at the time of chemotherapy. The American Society of Clinical Oncology recognizes and endorses this practice over hospital or outpatient clinical settings.

On the other hand, some oncologists send their patients to infusion centers, which are outpatient centers that treat a large number of patients on a daily basis. Registered nurses (RNs) administer chemotherapy, just like in an oncologist's office. They can address your concerns but the downside is that your doctor is not present, nor is your complete patient file. Most run efficiently, but because of the large number of patients treated on a daily basis, developing a personal relationship with patients is challenging. This type of relationship may or may not be important to you.

There is a higher probability of mistakes and infections in these centers. Some centers and physician's offices use a system of back-up nurses to confirm that the name and prescription for the chemotherapy drugs and blood transfusions is correct before beginning treatment in order to cut down on mistakes.

What Do Oncologists Expect From You?

During my interview with Dr. Fong, he provided some insight into the most common mistakes patients make that hinder their recovery. He explained that, unbelievably, patients do not always follow directions. They forget, do something else instead, or do nothing at all. In defense of patients, though, I have to say that the instructions for multiple prescriptions can be very complex even when written down. Memory or mental acuity might be impaired due to treatment.

When I was undergoing chemotherapy, my short-term memory function was less than stellar, primarily due to lack of sleep. Funny story—Our beloved Labrador retriever is notorious for hunting and eating whatever he can put his mouth around. When I got a phone call one night, I absent-mindedly left my bottle of steroid pills on the coffee table. I was about to prepare them for the following day of chemotherapy. After the phone call, the bottle was gone. If I did not take these pills, my chemotherapy schedule would surely have been interrupted. I hunted all over the house, only to find them intact on the kitchen floor. Thank goodness for tamper-proof bottle caps!

Remembering whether I had taken a drug five minutes prior was also challenging at times. I found that the best way to remedy the situation was to write everything down when given instructions and repeat it back. After taking scheduled medications check them off a daily list or have someone, help you at home.

I fully understand Dr. Fong's point of view regarding why following directions is so important. During chemotherapy, keeping the body's chemistry in balance is critical and if we fail to follow directions to the letter, it can be deadly.

Another concern is that we have limited appointment times with our oncologist and repeating information takes up valuable time when other new issues could be discussed. Your doctor is interested in how you are doing and wants to know. Leaving out something small that you believe is inconsequential can slow down treatment.

Perhaps it is human nature to only want to talk about our physical symptoms and the negative effects we suffer from when dealing with physicians. For some reason, we often fail to take into consideration our physician's personal philosophical views. We see them as a just a physician and their views deserve to be paid attention to for they can be just as important in the doctor-patient relationship.

When I asked the big question of what patients could do to make their treatments more successful, Dr. Fong's answer was unexpected. He replied, "Have a positive attitude and play an active role in your care." I thought it would be more complex.

I have always been the type of person that finds the good in everything. If the sun is not shining and someone says "What a gloomy day," my response typically is that I will make the best of it. Dr. Fong explained that a patient's positive attitude translates into far better outcomes. I am sure he is correct because he has seen thousands upon thousands of patients in his oncology practice. He knows who responded to treatment and who failed. We may not have the scientific data to support better outcomes from positive thinking but that does not mean it does not exist. How many of you have been in a room with strangers and tend to gravitate to the people who are smiling and have positive energy? Whatever they have, you want it too!

During cancer treatment, you want to encourage the professionals treating you to be the best at what they do. Medical professionals chose the field because they have a passion for helping people. We all know the saying "The squeaky wheel always gets taken care of first." Well, you very well might, but you may not endear yourself to the staff.

From my own experience in the chemotherapy room, the cheerful and friendly patients made it so much better for others feeling poorly or scared on their first day and subsequent days of chemotherapy. Hearing positive stories from patients on how they were doing or their many years of experience fighting cancer with Dr. Fong really helped. It gave me optimism, comfort, and made the time fly.

Cancer treatment is complex, and oncologists face the challenge of working in the capacity of a primary care physician during this time. Keep in mind that this is in addition to their typical duties. Oncologists also have the added responsibility of acting as a psychologist when dealing with patients. Some degree of counseling is unavoidable in the communication and interactions between our family, our oncologist and us in the decision-making process. We sometimes enlist the help of relatives or friends because we find it exceedingly difficult to make decisions and navigate the treatment process.

While at times as a cancer patient, we could have some physical limitations due to the disease and need assistance, it still is important for us to make the final decision on our care. Giving decision-making authority to someone else means not taking responsibility for our own fate.

As I mentioned earlier at the beginning of this guide, making hardcore final decisions regarding treatment is too difficult a task to delegate to someone else unless you are a child, in a coma, or suffer from mental illness or brain injury. If treatment is successful, everyone is happy. If treatment is unsuccessful, the decision-maker has to carry the guilt for the rest of their life. They probably would question whether the patient would still be alive if they had received some other form of treatment. Delegating this authority to someone else we could say is considered selfish and inconsiderate.

It is difficult for people to act appropriately when there is a life-threatening situation. When family dynamics enter into the equation, there is going to be a tug of war at times. Having the emotional and mental strength to deal with this is sometimes nearly impossible. It would be nice to run and hide, but we need to act like adults! I sympathize that under pressure, sometimes this is a lot to ask.

There are three emotional components to this. One is the shock of the cancer diagnosis. The second is not being emotionally ready to make decisions, and the third is the feeling of having to make a life-changing decision urgently.

Researchers in Germany have concluded that patients go into shock after diagnosis, and this frequently lasts for 3-6 months. In a recurrence, shock lasts only 2-4 weeks. If a patient is forced into taking a more active role in the healing process, he or she could end up feeling hopeless.[14] Some patients, while in shock, move into treatment quite quickly without exploring more options simply because they feel hopeless and it is easier to put their faith in one plan of attack. This is a profound effect. There is a huge psychological component involved in honoring a patient's own sense of timing, whether it is slow, fast or faster, but patients do need guidance to avoid the pitfalls of unwise decisions.

Throughout this process, it is your responsibility to bring up what you think would specifically benefit you and ask the opinion of your oncologist. Always trust your gut reaction; it can be incredibly important in assuring your survival. If something seems unsettling about their advice, ask more questions. If you still are not satisfied, there is nothing to lose by seeking a second or even third opinion. Go to another city, state or country to seek answers if necessary.

The oncologist you choose is going to be your greatest advocate during your care. He or she will follow your case for many years to come. It is important that you like, trust and appreciate them for the sacrifices they make in their personal lives to be on call 24/7 should you need them.

Chapter 7
Finding a Surgeon

Surgeons are skilled practitioners, but some are better than others. I interviewed a few surgeons experienced in cancer, and asked their opinion as to what makes a good surgeon. It was unanimous that most physicians trained in surgery have acquired the technical skills needed to operate. Having good judgment is what sets apart the good surgeons from the bad.

In all industries, the top 10% do the best work. If you are considering a surgeon, find out how their peers view their work and how many successful procedures they have performed. If your objective based on medical advice is to remove a tumor and one surgeon says he/she cannot, look for one who can. We all know our limitations. I never believe in no as an answer. When it comes to an operation, you want the best outcome and must find the most highly skilled surgeon for your particular situation.

When you hire a surgeon to perform an operation, you are entrusting them with your body and your life. When a tumor is involved, the best outcome is the careful extraction of the tumor and any cancerous or suspicious tissue around it on the first surgery.[12] Under a microscope during surgery, the surrounding tissue is analyzed. When no cancer is detected, the margins are considered clear of the disease. This is essential in keeping the cancer from spreading, although sometimes the operation alone has the potential to spread the cells by releasing them into the blood stream.

The sooner the tumor load is reduced by extracting the tumor, the easier it is for the body to fight the cancer. This is why sometimes surgery alone cures cancer. A second surgery results when margins are not cleared and can increase the risk of infection and surgery related injuries. The emotional and physical costs of repeated surgery are high.

Ask a surgeon how many surgeries they have performed relative to a specific cancer and how good the chances are of clearing the margins. At times, it has to do with where the cancer is located.

Chapter 8
What is Cancer?

Cancer comes in many different shapes and forms. No two patients or cancers are the same as both have biochemical differences. There are cancers of the blood, bone, lymph system, organs and skin. Every part of the human anatomy is subject to cancer in one form or another, whether it is a tumor or cells circulating in your blood and organs.

You cannot eat, drink, or breathe in cancer cells. The creation of cancer cells occurs inside the body when your immune system loses its ability to destroy them. Cancer is the result of a breakdown in the signaling process amongst cells. There are an estimated 50-100 trillion cells in the human body.[15] We produce and replace billions of cells per day. In an average adult, between 50 and 70 billion cells die each day due to programmed cell death. We have approximately 75 million cancer cells circulating in our body at any one time. The immune system keeps them under control so it does not develop into anything.

Cancer is the by-product of our cells acting abnormally because of damage. Our healthy cells produce DNA mutations daily, which can become cancer cells. Many cancers harbor multiple mutations, the majority of which most likely will have no significant effect on a cancer tumor's growth.

Cancer cells do not spread so much as they do not die at their programmed time. Cells have a normal life cycle and when death occurs, one healthy cell dies and two new ones are born. Out of those two cells, only one lives to replace the cell that has died, and if damaged in a particular way, these cells make bad copies of themselves. The result is that bad cells duplicate uncontrollably.

These bad cells are called oncocells, which turn into cancer cells. Oncocells sneakily enter the blood stream and coat themselves with fibrinogen glue and phlegm, making it impossible for the immune system to recognize them. They then stick together and form a colony of cells. This mass of cells embeds itself in a smooth muscle wall where they can access a blood supply and form a tumor.

Some cells start to go wrong at birth and do not send out strong enough signals that the immune system needs to kill them. Another example is cells with DNA damage from persistent chemical exposure through breathing, eating or drinking toxins. Cancer formation is a complex issue involving environmental, genetic, pharmaceutical and nutritional factors. Cancer can be in the body for 8-12 years before tumors form.

The presence of cancer denotes a failure, a mutation or a biological event. Once cancer is established, cancer cells go through specific growth cycles. The first cycle is the non-proliferating or resting stage. In the second cycle, cells synthesize ribonucleic acid (RNA) and protein. In the third cycle, sufficient RNA and protein develops and the cells progress to the DNA synthesis phase. DNA synthesis stops and RNA and protein synthesis continue in the fourth cycle. The final cycle involves the mitotic phase wherein cells divide and spread.

Any type of cancer, regardless from where it originates, can travel to distant parts of the body. This is called metastasis. Approximately 90% of all cancer deaths are the result of cancer spreading to other parts of the body through the lymphatic system and blood vessels to form additional tumors in other parts of the body.

Classification of Cancers

Cancers fall into the following categories:

Carcinoma. There are three different forms:

Basal cell carcinoma – This is the least dangerous of the skin cancers. It is visible on the surface of the skin, although it starts deep in the layers of the epidermal cells.

Squamous cell carcinoma – This is the second most common skin cancer. Squamous cell carcinomas are solid tumors of epithelial tissue (tissue forming a thin protective layer inside or outside the body). Tumors are found in layers of skin or over internal organs such as the stomach, uterus or testicles. Because epithelial tissue is composed of several different cell types in single sheets or layers, several different forms of carcinomas may present at the time of diagnosis.

Adenocarcinoma - These are quite common solid, malignant tumors of the epithelial tissue originating from cells in glands. The name of the cancer is based on the gland of origin, such as in lung cancer. Other organs of origination include the colon, breast, and prostate. Adenocarcinomas account for about

90-95% of all colorectal cancers and are common in non-small cell lung cancer.

Leukemia - There are four major types of leukemia, with acute being the most aggressive:

<u>Acute myeloid leukemia</u>
<u>Acute lymphoid leukemia</u>
<u>Chronic myeloid leukemia</u>
<u>Chronic lymphoid leukemia</u>

Leukemia is a form of cancer found in the blood circulatory system. The cells involved are abnormal T-or B-cells (types of WBCs) and sometimes the red blood cells (RBCs). Blood cells form within the bone marrow.

Lymphoma - There are two major categories of lymphomas:

<u>Hodgkin's lymphoma</u> (HL, was previously called Hodgkin's disease)
<u>Non-Hodgkin's lymphoma</u> (NHL)

Lymphoma affects cells in the lymphatic system, often creating solid tumors in the lymph nodes. There are 400-500 lymph nodes throughout the body. Flowing through the nodes is a lymph fluid composed of WBCs called disease-fighting T-cells and B-cells, along with proteins and fats. This fluid prevents the spread of infection by filtering out bad bacteria before it reaches our bloodstream.

Sarcoma - Sarcoma is a cancer of the connective tissues involving nerves, muscles, joints, bone, or blood vessels. There are over 50 subtypes of sarcomas and occur in either soft tissue or non-soft tissue. Their names originate from the tissue in which they began. Sarcomas can be found anywhere in the body and can be deep in the limbs. The American Cancer Society's key statistics state that common types of cancers are in soft tissue. Between 15-20% of all children's cancers are sarcomas. It is rarer in adults, with sarcomas accounting for only 1% of adult cancers.

Why Cancer?

Exposure to carcinogens along with "wear and tear" alters cells on a chromosomal level. Normally, our immune system takes them out so tumors and cancers do not have a chance to take hold.

Another way cancer develops is when normal genes turn bad by the breakdown of DNA. We subject our bodies to negative influences such as stress, lack of sleep, poor diet, toxic environmental pollution, chemical and radiation exposure, viruses, fungi and out-of-control free radicals, which are waste materials expelled by cells.

Mutant genes pass from one generation to another, causing tumor-suppressor genes to turn off. We know genes play a role in the initiation of cancer, but researchers are still looking for why it leads to cancer in some individuals and not others.

Breast, colon, ovarian and prostate cancers have a hereditary component. There are approximately 70 genes identified in carcinogenesis that become altered through naturally occurring circumstances and outside environmental exposures.

The International Cancer Genome Consortium (ICGC) was established in November of 2008. They coordinate large-scale projects to collect and categorize data in order to help researchers better understand what drives cancer. It is composed of research bodies in nine countries and the European Commission. Consortium members are collaborating on studies under the assumption cancer is not necessarily inherited. The "inheritance" gene simply increases the risk of developing cancer. The hope is treatments that target the mutations driving different types of cancer will be developed more quickly through this research. As of July, 2011, the ICGC announced its sixth major data release, generating a genomic database on more than 25,000 tumors for up to 50 types of cancer of clinical and societal importance across the globe.[16]

For incurable cancers, this exciting approach means that in the future, a wider range of drug combinations will be used because of pathology and mutation profiles. I am certain we will see the use of individualized cancer treatments within the next ten years gleaming better clinical outcomes and survival rates.

The ICGC also disclosed four gene mutations that cause CLL in different subgroups of patients. Sixty scientists in the Spanish Chronic Lymphocytic Leukemia Genome Consortium (LLGC) discovered the mutated genes when they sequenced the whole genome of normal and tumor cells of patients with CLL. I am hopeful more drugs will be developed in the near future that can target these mutations to treat CLL patients.

Carcinogens

It is very difficult to prove a cancer is the result of one or more specific carcinogens. Determining how long the exposure took place, how much of the carcinogen was absorbed into the body and what long-lasting effects caused cancer are supposition at best. Even so, the American Cancer Society promotes programs discouraging the use of cigarettes. These intense anti-smoking programs point out the high probability of developing lung cancer.

Another unknown is how a particular cancer will affect a patient in the long term. This is complicated because cancer has many variations and is unique to each patient. A biopsy and pathology report, along with blood work looking for tumor markers and genetic deviations allow for an educated guess as to how aggressive a cancer is and how likely it is to return.

Not all cancers have tumor markers that show up in blood tests. There are slow—and fast-growing cancers within every cancer type. Some people have one year or less in which to attempt therapy, whereas others have many years. Some people live into old age, whereas others are not as fortunate. The United States leads in the early discovery of cancer in its populations which results in better outcomes.

When newly diagnosed with cancer, it is important to understand your specific type of cancer and the options available for treatment. A physician cannot ever know with certainty whether a particular therapy will be entirely successful. In fact, when oncologists get creative and combine chemotherapy drugs outside of the norm, clinical trials may still be ongoing or do not even exist for the specific cancer in question. Take the example of when a patient fails a first time treatment for lung cancer with a traditional set of drugs. If it is subsequently determined that the cell mutations will likely respond to a drug commonly used for breast cancer treatment, along with two other drugs generally used for lung cancer, there will be no statistics regarding the likelihood of success of this unique treatment.

Oncologists have a fair amount of latitude in combinations of drugs they can try, so keep this in mind.

Clinical Trials and New Drugs

Doctors participate, read and write for medical journals and clinical research studies, confer with other physicians and find out about new drugs and protocols while attending conferences.

New research and publications are also available from clinical trials of new drugs. Clinical trials conducted with small groups of the population generally answer a specific research question or two. The criteria for acceptance into these groups are stringent. Pharmaceutical companies wanting to know whether their new drug is effective in treating certain cancers often fund these studies. New drugs, research and clinical trials for specific cancers undoubtedly save lives. New discoveries every day reveal the amazing work done by dedicated people worldwide.

You will find some studies by research universities that include a specific group of patients, anywhere from 10 to 1,000. Look for short—and long-term survival rates. The outcomes have a certain margin of error because a percentage of the patients do not follow the protocols or become too sick from the treatments to continue. Some cancer patients fail to meet certain qualifications and criteria for participating in trials.

It is helpful to know some studies also examine the placebo effect, meaning not all patients receive the actual drug(s) tested in the study. The effects of the particular drug in question can be more effectively determined with a placebo. People who volunteer for these studies provide a great service to humanity. By participating in these trials during a time of discomfort and suffering from cancer, they often save the lives of future generations by helping to determine the success of new drugs.

Busy practitioners, though, have limited time to read every relevant publication, attend conferences and learn about studies introducing new therapies. This is why it is so important to do research on your own, have a family member help or hire an outside consultant to advise you.

Every human body is unique and responds to medications and diseases in a different way. People have different genetic makeups and have had exposure to different levels of environmental pollutants and toxins. We may not all respond the same to a given therapy. People may have various pre-existing conditions, have received other medical treatments or drugs and have had better or worse nutrition throughout their lives. All these factors contribute to different outcomes in terms of cancer treatment success.

Oncologists in most states are bound to provide certain protocols and disclose certain information to their patients by their state medical laws and regulations. When in treatment, a patient may receive a cookie cutter treatment usually prescribed because of it having a high rate of success. For instance, they will administer the standard in the treatment of testicular cancer that is widely known to be very successful, rather than something that is more individualized.

Oncologists may be able to combine or switch certain drugs. Sometimes individual state laws, the FDA or insurance companies regulate the use of drugs and protocols, such as the amount of a drug used and treatment time span.

University research institutes and certain cancer centers that participate in research projects are often your best bet for obtaining treatments "off protocol" if necessary. Personalized drug therapy matched to one's genetic makeup or exact subcategory of cancer is practiced at these institutions. Keep in mind, though, if you become accepted into a clinical trial using an unproven drug, there are unknown risks, and uncertain outcomes. The good news is people have been cured in these programs.

A recent issue over the past few years is the controversy over drug companies taking new drugs to the market too soon without ample studies to prove their safety. In general, the birth of a new drug takes about 15 years. Laboratory studies take approximately 6-7 years. During the next 6-7 years, scientists test the drugs on people through clinical trials. They determine safety and if they can achieve the desired outcomes. The drug then undergoes further testing to see if it is superior to other treatments or placebos. Only one out of every five drugs passes this stage. After this stage, the results are submitted to the FDA for review. Most drugs go through a 10-18 month approval process. Some drugs are fast-tracked in only six months.

The controversy comes when the FDA allows drug companies to take their drug to the marketplace within as little as six months. These drugs go out into the marketplace without long-term research, meaning that the drug's safety is tested in the general population. Life-threatening situations and sometimes deaths occur, along with short-and long-term negative side effects. [17] Always ask physicians for the research support available for treatment protocols recommended to you.

CAM Published Studies

Because medical studies take place over a number of months or years and are quite costly, securing funds by the complementary alternative medicine, (CAM) or Eastern methods of healing are difficult to obtain. The National Cancer Institute (NCI) has historically remained the largest funding mechanism for cancer research and has a highly diversified program. The Office of Cancer

Complementary and Alternative Medicine (OCCAM) was created in 1998 due to the interest in CAM within the NCI. OCCAM coordinates and enhances activities of the NCI in CAM research. It researches the prevention, diagnosis, and treatment of cancer, along with cancer-related symptoms and side effects of conventional cancer treatments.

In fiscal year 2008, the NCI supported $121,264,507 in CAM-related research. This represents over 444 projects in the form of grants, cooperative agreements, supplements or contracts.[18] This is a fast-growing sector of research funding in the United States, taking place in cancer centers and at university research centers.[19]

This is very good news. The NCI funds and supports many ongoing studies in alternative medicine. Their position is that some treatments sound promising, but the safety and effectiveness of CAM treatments are questionable.[20] It is encouraging to know they are not opposed to exploring other therapies.

The best information you will find regarding CAM are in books, magazines and journals published and authored by the physicians and practitioners doing the work. They usually disclose their individual patient outcomes along with patient testimonials. CAM physicians generally have experience with medium to small patient populations who have cancer. Treatment approaches utilize various holistic medicines, therapies, nutraceuticals, herbs, minerals and vitamins.

The physicians practicing these methods do not usually have a large enough patient population to qualify their techniques as an accepted scientific or clinically-proven method for FDA approval. For them to conduct and publish studies is time-consuming and prohibitively expensive. Anecdotally, however, there are some impressive outcomes with patients experiencing cures, improved quality and extension of life.

The Johns Hopkins University Evidence-Based Practice Center in Baltimore, Maryland published a 321-page report in 2006 on "Multivitamin/Mineral Supplements and Prevention of Chronic Disease." They reviewed published literature from 1966 through February 2006 and queried experts from January 2005 through February 2006. Their conclusion was that multivitamin/mineral supplement use may prevent cancer in individuals with poor or suboptimal nutritional status in the United States.

In China, trial-examining individuals who were poorly nourished showed that supplementation combining beta-carotene, vitamin E and selenium reduced gastric cancer incidence and mortality, and overall cancer mortality. In a French trial, combined vitamin C, vitamin E, beta-carotene, selenium and zinc reduced cancer risk in men, but not in women. They found that selenium may help in cancer prevention overall.[21]

Nutrition and supplements can enhance immune function and help in fighting cancer by oxidizing cancer cells. When you limit glucose-producing foods that escalate cancer, cancer cell growth sometimes slows down. Good nutrition played a big role in keeping me strong in fighting cancer.

A study conducted in 2005 by Dr. Dean Ornish, a clinical professor of medicine at the University of California at San Francisco, involved 93 men with early-stage prostate cancer. The participants did not receive surgery and were split into two groups. One group was just under observation of their PSA number. The other group underwent a complete one year program that consisted of a vegetarian diet, particular supplements, physical exercise, stress management and one hour per week in a support group. At the conclusion of the study, the group that underwent a complete lifestyle change had an average tumor regression of 4%. Those who were in the observation group worsened, with patients receiving surgery, chemotherapy and radiation.[22]

Some experts believe taking large amounts of herbs and vitamins in high dosages may pose health risks, upsetting the natural metabolic balance in the body. I tend to agree when physician oversight is absent. Our body is a complex chemical machine and self-medicating with multiple supplements in large quantities without proper blood and urine analysis can have risks.

Every year in the CAM community, new cancer-fighting methods and treatments come into the marketplace for review. If traditional methods are thought of as ineffective or have only a small chance of success with a negative impact on quality of life, CAM is a viable option.

Chapter 9
Survival Rates

Survival rates is an important topic. We can talk about them all day long, but they are really just numbers that reflect how long people with certain cancers survive for a certain period. Even so, survival rates are important. The big question everyone wants an answer to when diagnosed is how is the cancer best cured? Patients also want to know the best-case scenario based on their physician's experience and survival statistics.

Survival rate statistics are calculated by following pools of patients who have received therapies and are still alive five years later (this reflects the five-year survival rate; if they follow patients for ten years, it would be a ten-year survival rate). Anyone who relapses before the target time is excluded from the survival statistics.

Information about age, general health, type of cancer and treatment successes based on modern medicine protocols are factored into these statistics. Calculating survival statistics involves hundreds of thousands of people. Overall survival rates can be separated into categories such as early and late diagnosis. There are many different types of cancers, and survival rates vary across types.

Survival rates are calculated in two formats. One is the percentage of people who have undergone treatment and are still surviving, cancer-free, after five years. Cancer-free means that the patient shows no signs of cancer. The second form of survival rates is the percentage of people who still have cancer, but whose disease is considered stable.

One interesting point is that the FDA considers a cancer treatment effective if it achieves a 50% or more reduction in tumor size for 28 days. Keep in mind that 28 days of treatment is not necessarily a cure for cancer or extension of life. It means there has been a temporary shrinkage.

Speaking for myself and other cancer survivors I know, we feel the day our physician declared us cancer free, we were cured. We have learned that remission is often used incorrectly by the public. The word remission should only be used involving certain leukemias because of high reoccurrence rates. Cure is used with all others. A cancer patient is cured of their disease as long as it is under control; which means there is no sign of the disease.

Information in categories such as age, general health, type of cancer and treatment successes based on modern medicine protocols factor into these statistics. Calculating survival statistics involves hundreds of thousands of people. Overall survival rates fall into categories of early and late diagnosis. There are many different types of cancers, and survival rates may vary.

In 2010, the National Institutes of Health (NIH) spent $290.3 million on cancer research. Their annual budget was an astounding $31.2 billion. The Centers for Disease Control and

Prevention (CDC) and the NCI published reports in 2011 indicating that death rates from all cancers in men and women continued to decline between the years 2003 and 2007.[23, 24] The CDC disclosed around 65% of cancer survivors lived at least 5 years after diagnosis, 40% lived 10 years or more and another 5% lived 25 years or longer. Cancer is considered primarily an "old person's disease," typically affecting individuals age 60 or older. I cannot help but be baffled by the amount of money spent on cancer research. We should have higher rates of survival in certain cancers by now.

One thing that is missing from these cumulative numbers is the amount of patients in the United States who have chosen to treat or cure their cancer through CAM treatments. There is no cumulative data tracked by any one large agency of CAM treatments worldwide due to lack of funding. Published research is needed to substantiate CAM techniques that work for cancer patients when traditional methods are not proving to be successful.

I have a painful personal example of when traditional therapies did not work and CAM might have been beneficial. A family member of mine had adenocarcinomas non-small cell lung cancer while writing this book. The time from diagnosis to the time of death was a little shy of four months. Treatment options for advanced lung cancer were limited. Through extensive research, it was evident little headway had been made in saving the lives of advanced adenocarcinomas non-small cell lung cancer patients. Rarely do these patients live long. My family and I feel deeply wounded by this event and it makes us determined more than ever to work harder toward advocating for more funds for early test detection for lung cancer.

People currently in the United States have many options for cancer treatment and have access to new drugs sooner than individuals do in other countries. With early diagnosis and treatment, this translates to cancer patients living longer in the United States than anywhere else in the world. The United States has the highest survival rates in 13 of 16 types of cancer. This is because of early detection. There is a 90% or higher survival rate with early detection of five cancers: skin melanoma, breast cancer, prostate cancer, thyroid cancer and testicular cancer. Europe only has one, testicular cancer.[25] In the United States, we have options in selecting physicians, tests, and protocols. Insurance companies, though, also have their say in what they are willing to pay for and who can provide your treatment.

There is a major shift occurring in research and how new cancer drugs are developed. I am hopeful that the road to manufacturing and approving these drugs becomes more efficient. Unfortunately, new drugs manufactured for the treatment of breast cancer fail in late-stage cancer 60-70% of the time based on clinical trials. The drugs proving marginally useful run around 30%.[26]

Researchers are using genetic information from patients and matching new drugs to the biological drivers of tumors. We know tumors have many mutations, and studies are validating that patients respond better when targeting specific mutations on tumor cells. Thus, we are seeing more support for individualized treatment protocols designed for each patient.[27]

Studies have shown that patients who receive drugs that target their specific mutations live longer. Unfortunately, these treatments are not offering any cures. Most of these studies are mostly taking place in research facilities. However, starting in 2010, routine genetic profiling of tumors was being offered. Massachusetts General Hospital and MD Anderson Cancer Center are among the institutions in the United States offering

genetic profiling of tumors now and in the future other institutions will follow due to plummeting costs.[28]

In 2011, over 800 drugs designed just to target mutations are
in various stages of development. The additional costs involved
are requirements by the FDA to develop companion diagnostic
tests that are separate from drug approval.

I do not believe a patient should be stuck on a number for
survival. We all are unique in our thinking, beliefs, culture, and
body chemistry. In addition, these large statistical banks of information include many different types of cancer therapies. For
instance, the survival rates I found for CLL did not apply to me
because I had not yet undergone any traditional therapies the
survival rates addressed. The important thing to remember is
statistics are just one way to measure outcomes. Cancer drugs
are mixed in many different combinations and have more or less
success with each individual. Statistics reflect patient outcomes
of certain drug combinations used. At best, survival statistics
can serve as a barometer and certainly cannot predict your own
outcome.

Chapter 10
Complementary and Alternative Medicine

Patients can choose treatment protocols for cancer that involve a combination of traditional Western medicine drugs and therapies. We also have the option of using natural, complementary, alternative, eastern and holistic medicines.

When surveyed, 70% of people diagnosed with cancer were not satisfied with the three choices offered by conventional Western medicine. We all know what these are: chemotherapy, radiation and surgery. Some cancer patients believe that alternative therapies support chemotherapy and radiation treatments and enhance overall general health.[29]

There is great deal of debate as to the value of these more non-traditional methods of treatment. In 2011, a study published by MD Anderson Cancer Center determined that out of 309 patients surveyed, 52% used one or more alternative supportive treatments. The most frequently used were vitamins (70%) and herbal products (26%).[30]

Interestingly, there was no statistically significant association between the use of CAM and quality of life as perceived by the patients. Perhaps this was because it was difficult to distinguish between the factors that contributed to poor quality of life in later stages of cancer, especially when traditional therapies such as chemotherapy and radiation were used simultaneously. It is my opinion it would be difficult to survey exactly how patients felt because health status can change from day to day. Also of interest in this study was that 23% of the patients neglected to disclose their CAM use to their physicians. Lack of disclosure is a common trend.

A study conducted by Emory University Rollins School of Public Health found that at the beginning of treatment, 56% of prostate cancer patients used supplements and did not disclose use to their physicians.[31]

There is a large disconnect between patients and their physicians concerning CAM. The big question to ask is whether supplements interfere with chemotherapy, or whether they enhance patient outcomes. Patients may also pay for such treatments privately and not disclose it to their physicians. The challenge when taking supplements is knowing which ones conflict with traditional medicine and which ones help with toxicity. It takes an expert to determine this.

Chapter 11
Blood and the Immune System

Trained professionals in medicine and science live in the world of medical and technical terminology. Most of us have difficulty understanding this new vocabulary. I, for one, had quite a time of it! However, because my belief is so strong in the research and data supporting how integral healthy blood and the immune system is for good health, fighting cancer, and in recovery, I am compelled to cover this topic. It is important to know how it fits into the big picture so you have a better understanding of what is happening to your body during treatment.

Common Blood Tests

Diagnostic blood tests are vital for monitoring your progress during treatment. Blood is drawn in different quantities for various tests. Blood is the "mirror" of overall health. When viewing it under a microscope, it is alive with movement!

You most likely will have weekly blood draws while undergoing treatment. I have always tracked blood results with a natural curiosity and have learned how to interpret most reports.

Our blood tests are an excellent indicator of areas needing improvement. An example would be a case in which RBCs are low, resulting in a diagnosis of anemia. A physician might advise you to eat more vegetables with iron, or to use iron supplements. If hemoglobin and blood platelets are low, you should be cautioned to avoid injury due to potential excessive bleeding or bruising, along with possible fatigue.

CBC/Chemistry Blood Panel

The CBC is a standard test that examines the levels of various components of the blood. When certain components are out of the normal range, either high or low, it may raise a red flag. I will only cover the basic CBC panel as it pertains to you as a cancer patient. This is the one test that will most often be done by your oncologist.

Here is an explanation of the standard CBC lab report. It will help you learn how to read and interpret results.

• **White blood cell (WBC)** counts—This measures the number of WBCs in a cubic millimeter of blood. Increases in counts may denote the flu, infection, inflammation or cancer. Decreases could be related to medications or minor viral infections.

• **Red blood cell (RBC)** counts—This measures the number of RBCs in a cubic millimeter of blood. Decreases in counts may denote illness, fatigue, shortness of breath, paleness in color, dizziness or may be due to medications. An increase in numbers can cause headaches, flushing and disturbed vision.

- **Hemoglobin**—Measures the oxygen carried to the tissues. Decreases in counts may denote cancer, anemia, fatigue, shortness of breath, paleness in color, dizziness or may be due to medications. Increases could be from dehydration, living in high altitudes, bone marrow disease or other illness.

- **Hematocrit**—This is the percent of cellular components in the blood as compared to the fluid or blood plasma. Used in diagnosing anemia. A decrease is always seen with a decrease in hemoglobin. Increases are associated with dehydration.

- **Mean corpuscular volume (MCV)**—This is a measure of the average RBC volume. Increases can be from medications, deficiencies in vitamin B12 and folic acid. Decreases are associated with anemia.

- **Mean corpuscular hemoglobin (MCH)**—This is a measure of the average mass of hemoglobin per RBC. Increases can be from medications, deficiencies in vitamin B12 and folic acid. Decreases are seen in anemia.

- **Mean corpuscular hemoglobin concentration (MCHC)**—This is a measure of the concentration of hemoglobin in a given volume of packed RBCs. Increases can be from medications, deficiencies in vitamin B12 and folic acid. Decreases are seen in anemia. In addition, MCHC is elevated in spherocytosis and pernicious anemia.

- **Red blood cell distribution width (RDW)**—This shows the degree of consistency in the size of the RBCs.

Increases are seen in anemia, alcohol abuse and some cancers. Decreases are associated with anemia and rheumatoid arthritis.

• **Platelets**—Platelets are cellular fragments made in the bone marrow that are necessary for the blood to clot. With counts as low as 50,000, people can survive without the threat of excessive internal bleeding. Increases in platelet counts are due to strenuous activity, illness, infection, inflammation, cancer, or spleen removal and can cause blood clots to form. Decreases can be from cancer or other illness and can cause inflammation.

• **Mean platelet volume (MPV)**—This shows how large platelets are. The size denotes whether there are any issues with platelet production in the bone marrow. Low levels could be due to bone marrow cancer.

• **Lymphocytes (LYMPHS)**—Lymphocytes are divided into B (bone marrow matured) and T (thymus matured). They regulate antibody production and are responsible for immune response. An increase can be due to cancer, serious illnesses or the flu. Decreases can be found from viral illness, steroids, medications, or anemia.

• **Monocytes (MO)**—Monocytes eat foreign invaders and protect against infection. They increase with chronic infections, inflammation, illness and cancer. A decrease can be due to cancer and bone marrow malfunction.

• **Granulocytes (GR)**— Granulocytes protect against infection and come from the bone marrow. They increase with infections, inflammation, illness and cancer. A decrease can also be present with cancer.

- **Neutrophils (NEUT)**—Neutrophils are the most common of WBCs. They increase with infections, spread of cancer, inflammation, medications, obesity and smoking. Decreases are associated with cancer medications and illness.

- **Eosinophils (EOS)**—Eosinophils are important in fighting infections but are present only in a very small percentage in the blood. They increase with infection, allergies and cancer. Decreases are due to stress, certain medications, and allergies.

- **Basophils (BAS)**—Basophils contain granules and are the least numerous of leukocytes. They are related to mast cells. They contain histamine, so an increase is generally due to allergies, inflammation, cancer and radiation exposure.

Other tests examine mineral levels, vitamin levels (particularly vitamins D and B12), sugar levels, indicators of possible infection, hormone levels (in certain cancers), tumor markers, proteins, and immunoglobulins. WBC counts fall into many different categories and can have different meaning depending upon the type of cancer you have.

Blood

When we understand the mechanics of the blood, the immune system, and how all organs and cells in our bodies interconnect for optimal health, we are better equipped to make the right decisions in terms of our health care options. Unfortunately, with cancer, making the wrong treatment decisions can be life threatening, thus weakening the immune system and causing setbacks. Chemotherapy and radiation treatments are harsh because they cannot distinguish between killing good and bad cells.

Environmental toxins, genetic mutations, poor nutrition, stress, illness, emotional issues and lack of sleep also contribute to a poor functioning immune system. Think of the immune system as a massive bodyguard shielding us from harm. It will reward us with many trouble-free, healthy years when it is efficient, or it can cause major issues when it is dysfunctional. We do not want to harm the important organs and cells that make up the immune system. Organ failure is not an option. Keep a watchful eye on blood test results, specifically the WBC panel. White and red blood cell counts can fluctuate drastically, possibly triggering changes in hemoglobin and platelet counts. These play vital roles in cancer treatment and recovery.

Once diagnosed with cancer and enrolled in a treatment program, blood draws become a common occurrence. Blood labs on occasion do make mistakes, so if something comes back suspicious or worrisome, have the test done again. There is no sense in taking prescribed medications or undergoing a procedure needlessly due to false positive test results.

Blood work is very telling as to how well the immune system is holding up under a treatment protocol for cancer. It also reveals improvements or regressions in health. The immune system really is an amazing and complex system involving many different organs and cells in our bodies. The immune system deciphers differences between the body's own unique cells and foreign cells.

The two primary lymphoid organs important in the immune system are the thymus gland and the spleen, where active immune cells develop and some mature. Other lymphoid organs are the bone marrow, lymph nodes, tonsils and appendix. These organs and cells act as a filtration system and are the backbone of our immune defenses.

The Thymus Gland

The thymus gland is located between the breastbone and the heart. The thymus produces T-cells, also called natural killer T-cells. Natural killer T-cells are lymphocytes, a form of WBC. Their most important role is destroying cancer and cells infected by a virus. The thymus also produces a hormone called tymosin, which encourages lymphocyte production. By age 21, the thymus is fully functional with an abundance of T-cells. By age 40, it shrinks and is less effective.

The Spleen

The spleen is about the size of a clenched fist and is located in the upper left area of the abdomen close to the stomach under the rib cage. It is the largest lymphoid organ in the human body and filters all the blood in our body every 90 minutes, holding between 30 and 40 mL of blood. It looks for foreign cells such as bacteria and old RBCs in need of replacement. If you exercise hard, it releases blood into your system to compensate for any blood loss in other parts of your body. People can live without a spleen (accidental or purposeful removal), but immune system functioning is slightly compromised. In some cancers, the spleen enlarges and expands into the abdominal cavity, causing it to be at high risk for injury or rupture.

Bone Marrow

Well-functioning bone marrow is vital to our overall health. It is a soft, sponge-like tissue in the center of our bones. Bone marrow produces new white and red blood cells important for immune functioning and platelets responsible for clotting our blood. RBCs mature and enter our bloodstream, whereas WBCs mature later.

Stem cells are responsible for branching off and becoming different, specialized types of cells. They come from bone marrow, as well as embryos and amniotic fluid. Master cells, also called daughter cells, have the ability to duplicate and become either new stem cells or specialized cells with specific functions, such as blood cells, brain cells, heart muscle and bone. Stem cells are unique and we are now beginning to understand their full potential in the renewal of organs; the growth of new ones, and how stem cells affect long-term good health.

In some cancers, the bone marrow can cease to function properly due to an overabundance of cancer cells. This can upset the natural balance between red and white blood cells and platelets, which wreaks havoc on the body. Any imbalance can create a multitude of symptoms and illnesses.

Lymph Nodes

The main priority of lymph nodes is to filter lymph fluids before returning to the blood. They also contribute to immunity by providing WBCs called lymphocytes and macrophages when needed. The lymphatic system consists of approximately 400-500 nodes in various clusters located in the jaw, chin, neck, armpits, chest, abdomen, pelvis and groin.[32] Lymph nodes produce fluids that circulate, drain and distribute nutrients and collect waste. Lymph fluids circulate when we move around, contract our muscles or get body massages.

In certain cancers such as those of the lymphatic system, the lymph nodes become hard and enlarged because of cancer cell infiltration. In some illnesses, they temporarily enlarge while the body is fighting infection.

White Blood Cells

The normal WBC count range is 3,300 to 8,700 per microliter (mcL), although this can vary from one blood lab to another. If your neutrophil count falls below 1,000 mcL, this could indicate cancer or the effects of cancer drugs. A low neutrophil count may increase the chances of developing a bacterial infection and is called neutropenia. Conversely, neutrophils over 8,000 mcL are very high and could signal cancer or another health issue.

In cancer, the first blood counts to drop are usually those related to WBCs because they have the shortest lifespan. If the bone marrow is not able to make new ones fast enough, their counts will drop after a few days of therapy.

When a patient is receiving chemotherapy, physicians will sometimes recommend medication to stimulate WBC growth factors from your bone marrow, lower the dose of chemotherapy or stop it altogether until the counts recover. Physicians will also recommend their patients advise them the minute they think they are getting the flu or an infection. Getting treatment immediately can lessen the degree of infection and symptoms and can ultimately be lifesaving. Cancer patients can die from infections because of low immune function.

When WBCs exceed 8,700 per mcL, it could be due to cancers involving the blood and bone marrow. The excessive production of WBCs is called leukocytosis. Examples would be multiple myeloma, lymphoma or leukemia.

Lymphocytes

Lymphocytes are specialized forms of WBCs that originate in the bone marrow and travel to the spleen, lymph nodes and thymus gland. They split into two groups: B-lymphocytes and T-lymphocytes. Those destined to specialize as B-cells travel in and out of the lymph nodes and the spleen. These cells mature into plasma cells, producing antibodies against antigens (foreign matter in the blood). They have a short life span and do not play a major role in fighting cancer.

Lymphocytes that become T-cells travel via the blood to the thymus gland where they mature. T-lymphocytes then split into two groups: helper T-cells and natural killer T-cells. These travel throughout the circulatory fluid system of the body, finding bacteria and viruses. They are the body's most potent immune responder for cancer prevention and control. It takes several days for lymphocytes to identify and attack foreign invaders. These cells can live for hours, weeks, months or years. In some blood cancers, they do not die as they should, and crowd out the bone marrow. This will show up in a blood test as an abnormally high WBC count,

Red Blood Cells

RBCs originate in the bone marrow and account for about 40-45% of our blood volume. They contain hemoglobin and make a protein that helps distribute oxygen from the lungs to the rest of the tissues in the body. The cells then transfer carbon dioxide from our tissues back to the lungs where excess carbon dioxide is exhaled. Hemoglobin regulates the amount of carbon dioxide throughout the body. It also contains iron.

There are approximately 25 trillion RBCs in our bodies. They die at about two million cells per second, and new cells are formed approximately every 120 days. A normal range is 4,000-6,000 mcL. Hematocrit is usually between 38-48% of the blood. In cases of cancer, low RBC counts could be due to bone marrow suppression. Some chemotherapy and radiation treatments can also affect RBC levels. On a blood lab test, look for low levels of RBCs, hemoglobin and hematocrit. Low values are associated with anemia.

The Complement System

The complement system protects us from bacterial infections and involves as many as 60 different circulating proteins in our blood and tissues. These are produced and dispersed by the liver, WBCs, and gastrointestinal and genitourinary (genital and urinary) tracts. Specific cells have receptors (proteins) on their surface to identify antigens.

Antigens have two different pathways in which they work. One is the *classical*, which requires an army of antibodies to attach themselves to bacteria and embed themselves into cell walls, creating a hole and ultimately causing cell death. The second is the *alternative*, in which rings of proteins in a cell are created, making a hole that then bursts.

Hemoglobin

Hemoglobin is extremely important as a component of RBCs. It carries iron-containing oxygen to the tissues. Normal levels seen in blood lab reports are 12-16 grams per deciliter (g/dL) for adult females and 14-18 g/dL for adult males. In some cancers and treatment protocols, these levels can drop to abnormally low levels and can cause difficulty breathing, increased fatigue, heart palpitations, chest pain, and the feeling that one's legs are heavy while walking. These symptoms are due to less oxygen circulating in the blood, causing the body to work harder to deliver oxygen throughout the body. If the levels drop too low, blood transfusions might be needed. For every pint of blood, the hemoglobin level will raise one g/dL. For example, it would move up from 6 g/dL to 7 g/dL. When hemoglobin levels are high, this may indicate bone marrow malfunction, but not necessarily cancer. Another cause of low hemoglobin is anemia, which could be induced by receiving chemotherapy or from cancer itself.

Platelets

Platelets are fragments of cells and come from bone marrow stem cells. They perform a clotting function to stop bleeding. Normal counts are 150,000-300,000 per cubic millimeter of blood (CuMM) in adults. Low levels can be a sign of blood cancers. If the platelet count drops below 50,000 CuMM, there is a high risk of internal bleeding or excessive external bleeding if wounded. Some people experience bruising and/or a rash of small purple or red dots on the body. Cancer treatments can also cause low platelet counts. Platelet numbers typically recover once treatment has stopped for a short time. In certain cancers, stem cell transplantation is an option to improve bone marrow function, but is not without major risks.

Chapter 12
The Phagocytic Family

There are four types of phagocytic cells. They are important in destroying dead and foreign cells: monocytes, neutrophils, eosinophils and basophils.

Monocytes

Monocytes are the largest of the WBCs. They are produced in the bone marrow and half of them can be later found in the spleen. Their function is to attack bacteria or viruses. They make up 1-3% of the WBCs in the body. When there is an increase in their numbers, you could be fighting off an infection or have inflammation.

Neutrophils

Neutrophils are the first line of defense against infection. They come from our bone marrow and go after bacteria and foreign debris. They make up more than half of the WBCs in the peripheral circulation of the blood. There are two types: band (immature) and segmented (mature). A bacterial infection causes the body to make more neutrophils, which results in a higher than normal WBC count.

Basophils

Basophils originate in the bone marrow and are created by stem cells. Their count in blood is usually very low. They contain large amounts of histamine, serotonin and heparin. They become elevated in instances of an active infection or allergic reaction. This could be from a bee sting, anaphylaxis brought on by a drug interaction, bronchial asthma or hives.

Eosinophils

Eosinophils are 1-3% of the WBC count. They are involved in responding to parasitic invasion, viral infections, destroying cancer cells and are involved in allergic responses. Eosinophil counts will be high when the body experiences any of the above circumstances.

Chapter 13
Antibodies

Macrophages

Macrophages are cytokines (interleukins, interferons and growth factors). They are WBCs that play a major role in cell immunity, growth, development, cell death and getting rid of worn out cells and other debris. They have a positive or negative effect in our body depending on how they are working. In the instance of cancer, they fight off cancer or malfunction along with other cells and get in the way of warding off disease. Macrophages look for foreign invaders giving off antigens, and if our cells are working properly, they seek and destroy invaders such as pathogens, viruses, fungi, bacteria and parasites, which lower our immune system defenses.

When the immune system recognizes drugs, pollens, insect venoms, chemicals in foods, malignant cells and foreign tissue, it naturally reacts in complex ways. For example, in an organ transplant or blood transfusion, it recognizes foreign material and works to "reject" the organ or blood transfusion. Rejection is the way our body attempts to protect us from getting sick, fever-ish, or even from dying.

B-cells secrete antibodies called immunoglobulins and gamma globulins. They respond to specific antigens like bacteria, viruses or toxins. These proteins each respond and bind to a specific an-tigen (bacteria, virus or toxin). This binding disables the chemi-cal action of the toxin.

As they recognize an antigen as a foreign invader, antibodies stimulate the body to continue making more antibodies for protec-tion. Through this mechanism, the body becomes immune to the antigen and wards off illness. Immunoglobulins are blood proteins and not good tumor marker indicators. In some cancers affecting the bone marrow, a person may have too much of one type of immu-noglobulin circulating in the blood. Measuring the levels over time during a treatment protocol shows how well a patient responds to a particular cancer treatment.

Immunoglobulins

There are five classes of immunoglobulins in the human body. They assist in directing the right immune response for each kind of foreign invader they encounter. They are as follows:

Immunoglobulin A (IgA)

The IgA molecule can be secreted across a mucous membrane. Because of this, it can defend against infections involving the respiratory system and the intestinal tract. IgA counts will be high in cases of cancer such as myeloid myeloma.

Immunoglobulin D (IgD)

IgD is the most common antibody bound to inactive B and T-cells. Its purpose is to trigger an immune response. Decreases are associated with CLL.

Immunoglobulin E (IgE)

IgE is involved in allergic reactions such as asthma, hay fever and hives. It can trigger inflammation from histamines released after attacks of pathogens. Increases may also indicate the cancer IgE myeloma.

Immunoglobulin G (IgG)

IgG makes up around 80% of the antibodies in the blood. It is the most efficient in neutralizing toxins. It is decreased in the cancers IgA myeloma and CLL.

Immunoglobulin M (IgM)

The body produces IgM the first time the immune system is exposed to a new foreign agent. Ninety-nine percent of anti-cancer antibodies generated by the immune system are of the IgM subclass.

Chapter 14
Hormones

Throughout our lives, hormones play a vital role in chemical regulation and balancing our bodies. Hormones send chemical messages to our organs and tissues and orchestrate metabolic processes by creating changes in our cells. Without hormones, our bodies are open to infection, fatigue, osteoporosis, skin problems, coronary heart disease, sexual dysfunction, thyroid problems, fertility issues and disease. Cancer can also be a possible consequence.

If you undergo chemotherapy or radiation, your hormones suffer along with your immune system. Steroids and corticosteroids (components of adrenaline) used to help keep your body from rejecting the chemotherapy drugs also upset the body's natural balance and cause excessive inflammation. Steroids can raise glucose levels, which suppresses the immune system and make you more vulnerable to illness during treatment. I was told to drink plenty of fluids to help flush out my system and to stay out of public places when my immune system was low (indicated by low WBC counts).

Many cancerous tumors or organs affected by cancer have hormone dominance issues. This is particularly true in breast and prostate cancers. It is important to know what your levels are prior to treatment as a baseline. In breast cancer, for instance, if a patient is estrogen positive and her estrogen levels are extremely high, some physicians will check and compare levels once treatment is finished.

As we age, our hormone levels change and we become more prone to disease and the effects of aging. Environmental toxins can also convert into xenoestrogens, which play with the body's balance of hormones.

Below is a list of human hormones important in a discussion of cancer.

- Estrogen (composed of estradiol, estrone and estriol)
- Progesterone
- Testosterone
- DHEA
- Thyroid
- Androgens-(DHT)-composed-of androstenedione-and-di hydrotestosterone
- Melatonin
- Cortisol and Pregnenolone

Estrogen

Estrogen is the most powerful of all the hormones. Interestingly enough, while estrogen is usually thought of in regard to women's health, both men and women have estrogen. Women produce most of their estrogen in their ovaries, whereas men go through a chemical process involving an enzyme called aromatase that transforms testosterone into estradiol. Estradiol is one of the three steroid hormones in the estrogen family. The other two are estrone and estriol.

While proper estrogen levels have a multitude of health benefits, when your levels are too high it can have negative repercussions. Elevated levels of estrogen are linked to breast enlargement in young males. Men can experience weight gain, prostate enlargement and loss of libido.[33] Dr. John Lee, an internationally renowned pioneer and expert in natural hormones stated men with long-term exposure to high estrogen levels over 30 picograms per milliliter (pg/ml) of serum can signal excess aromatase enzyme activity triggering prostate enlargement and prostate cancer.[34] A study published in 2006 confirmed that men with benign prostate enlargement or prostate cancer have higher blood estrogen levels and often have low free testosterone in their blood.[35]

Georgetown Lombardi Comprehensive Cancer Center discovered that one type of estrogen in a man's body might increase the risk of developing prostate cancer, but another type might protect it.[36] What we do not know at this time is whether it is the body's natural estrogenic properties that are protective or whether outside influence from hormone-mimicking substances factor in. In another study, it was determined that estrogens directly affect prostate cells and modulate their biological functions.[37]

There is a hypothesis that hormone therapy might contribute to prostate cancer in men, but there is little research support for this premise. Low levels of testosterone are associated with a greater risk of aggressive prostate cancer. Prostate cancer was one of the top ten cancers in men in the United States in 2006, with prostate cancer at the top of the list for all races.

High levels of estrogen in females can lead to the early development of sexual characteristics such as early menses around 12 years old and breast development as young as 7-8 years of age, which is five years earlier than the established norm.[38] It can also lead to breast cancer in women. Estrogen dominance exists when there are low levels of progesterone to counterbalance estrogen levels.

Biopsies on breast tissue have found that the percentage of breast cancers testing hormone-receptor positive predominately for estrogen rather than progesterone in premenopausal women was around 50%. In postmenopausal women, it can be up to 70%. As discussed earlier, estrogen is a precursor to cancer growth.

The big question is how we end up with estrogen or progesterone dominance. One reason for the elevation of estrogen is the presence of xenoestrogens, which alter our normal estrogen levels. Think of xenoestrogens as manmade toxins. They enter our bodies through our food, water, cleaning products, cosmetics, and the air we breathe. Food and drink containers made of plastics containing polychlorinated biphenyls (PCBs) are released into our food and water.

It has become increasingly evident that consuming meat contributes to estrogen dominance. Farm animal feed contains hormones designed to increase body size and weight. Ranchers routinely use low levels of antibiotics in feed and water to promote faster growth and prevent infections. Humans then ingest these hormones, which increase their own hormone levels.[39]

Eating fish can also contribute to the problem, because the fish we eat have PCBs. These PCBs come from farm-fed fish that receive food with PCBs in them. Chemicals such as mercury circulate in the air and then end up at the bottom of the ocean floor. Fish eat off the bottom of the ocean floor and ingest the mercury.

Progesterone

Progesterone is produced only in females. The most important role progesterone plays in the body is to balance and oppose estrogen. When estrogen levels are abnormally high and progesterone levels are low, it can upset the natural balance and lead to cancer. When estrogen becomes the dominant hormone, the result is increased body fat, salt and fluid retention, breast stimulation (tenderness and enlargement) and an increase in the mucous membrane (the thickness) of the uterus.[40,41] When xenoestrogens enter the body and boost estrogen levels, the risk of breast and endometrial cancers increase.

In 2002, a study conducted by The Women's Health Initiative followed 16,000 women taking hormone replacement therapy over a five-year period. The therapy combined estrogen and progestin. Researchers concluded that conjugated equine estrogens (0.625 mg/d) plus medroxyprogesterone acetate (2.5 mg/d in 1 tablet) or placebo caused a small increase in the risk of invasive breast cancer and larger, more advanced cancers. There also was an increase in heart attacks, strokes and blood clots. There were decreases in broken hips and colorectal cancers.[42, 43]

We should recognize that the hormones used in this study were synthetic, pharmaceutical grade hormones rather than bio identical hormones that are derived from concentrated soy and yam. Premarin is derived from horse urine estrogens and was approved by the FDA in 1942.[44] Prempro is a horse urine-derived estrogen and a synthetic progestin. Neither of these hormones are identical in structure.[45] There is no question this study gave compelling evidence against the use of synthetic, pharmaceutical grade hormones for extended periods of time.[46]

Would the outcomes have been different if this study used natural progesterone and natural estriol? I researched "natural" bio-identical hormone replacement therapy to answer this question. The protective element of progesterone has been studied by following 1,083 women with a history of difficulty becoming pregnant.[47] Researchers found that infertile women with progesterone deficiency had a pre-menopausal breast cancer risk 540% greater than women who were infertile due to non-hormonal causes.[48] What I find more astonishing is that women with progesterone deficiency were 1,000% more likely to die from all types of cancers. This strongly suggests natural progesterone protects women against breast cancer.[49]

One of the biggest controversies over the past 10 years has been this difference in outcomes between using bio-identical estrogen, progesterone and other hormones versus synthetic hormones. Bio-identical hormones are chemically identical to the ones produced in the body, and the body cannot tell the difference. The body metabolizes and excretes them in the same way as those naturally produced in the body. By law, these hormones are mandated to be compounded and sold from a compounding pharmacy in the United States, and are usually available by prescription from your doctor. Marketers of bio-identical hormones say their products have these advantages over standard hormone therapies: Bio-identical hormones are derived from plant chemicals, not synthesized in a laboratory. Some FDA-approved products (Estrace, Climara and Vivelle-Dot patches, and Prometrium natural progesterone) proclaim they are derived from plants also.

Bio-identical hormones are produced in doses and forms very different from those in FDA-approved products. Some bio-identical hormone products are available without a prescription, but most require one.

You can go through a compounding pharmacy for many nonstandard combinations. Compounding pharmacies specialize in customizing medications to an individual, such as when the patient is unable to swallow solids or is allergic to a binding agent in a tablet. Products from compounding pharmacies have not been subject to the same rigorous quality assurance standards as commercially available hormonal preparations, but may be just as good in quality. Some bio-identical hormone products are available without a prescription, but most require them.

There are small studies showing bio-identical progesterone does not induce estrogen-stimulated breast cell proliferation.[45] I have not been able to find a single randomized trial (the gold standard of medical research) comparing pharmaceutical grade and bio-identical hormones and the effect they have on women's health. The jury is out as far as I can tell. You should discuss with your physician what they consider safe for use. Regular blood tests to monitor levels of progesterone and other hormones is required if you decide to use them.

Testosterone

Men have ten times more testosterone than women do. Testosterone is a vital hormone with levels that peak during youth and decline with age. In men, it is produced by the testicles. When there is a loss of testosterone, it affects the diameter of blood vessels, libido, bone and muscle mass. It also affects cardiovascular and emotional health.

A risk factor of low testosterone in men is the development of metabolic syndrome and Type 2 Diabetes. After age 40, men experience andropause, or the natural and gradual loss of testosterone. Testosterone levels generally fall 0.4-1.2% per annum because of normal aging.[50]

The New England Research Institutes in Massachusetts conducted a study of men between the ages of 45 and 80. Researchers found that American men are experiencing a substantial decline in testosterone that does not seem to be attributable to health or lifestyle characteristics such as smoking or obesity. It also is greater in magnitude than the cross-sectional declines in testosterone typically associated with age.[51]

Hypogonadism is when the sex glands produce little or no hormones. In 2006, it was disclosed that the overall prevalence of this condition was approximately 39% in men aged 45 and older. Recent estimates are that 13 million men in the United States experience testosterone deficiency and fewer than 10% receive treatment for it.[52] I suspect the numbers are much higher because men do not frequent doctor's offices as much as women and when they do, testosterone levels are probably not on their list of things to check.

A recent pooled analysis was done in 2010 sponsored by Life Extension magazine involving subscribed members of their Life Extension Foundation examining a total of 7,619 men. Free testosterone blood tests uncovered an epidemic of testosterone deficiency in Life Extension members. Only 4.2% of the men in the study had high optimal free testosterone blood levels. Another 9.6% were in the mid-range, at 15-22 pg/ml. The big question here is what caused 86% of the men in this group to have less than 15 pg/ml of free testosterone? [53]

Dr. Leigh Erin Connealy, a Board-Certified Family Practice and Wellness Medical doctor says she finds low levels of free testosterone to be common in men in their 30's. It is possible that one of the factors contributing to low testosterone levels is the presence of xenoestrogens, which, as discussed earlier, disrupt the normal levels of hormones in the body. They can increase estrogen levels and upset the natural balance of testosterone.

It is not something getting much press, but ask the wives or girlfriends of these men with low testosterone, and they probably would confirm their significant others suffer from one or more of the symptoms accompanying andropause. Symptoms include fatigue, change in personality affecting attitude and mood, loss of sex drive and energy or less physical agility.

Testosterone deficiency shows up in other ways, such as decrease in body hair, muscle mass or osteoporosis. Testosterone deficiency is similar to menopause in women. When high levels of estrogen are found in men, there can be harmful effects on the prostate gland. In terms of men's overall longevity, studies supported by a 20-year follow-up showed that men with low testosterone had a 33% greater chance of dying over an 18-year time period than those with higher levels. Some of these individuals died from diseases such as cardiovascular, diabetes and respiratory conditions. [50] Some physicians recommend that low testosterone levels be increased via supplements. Gels, pellets, and creams are available through qualified physicians.

DHEA

DHEA is a "precursor" hormone, one that the body can convert to over 50 essential hormones including testosterone, estrogen, progesterone and cortisone. DHEA levels play a role in immune functioning and in longevity. We have high levels of the steroid hormone DHEA when we are young, and levels drop as we age. By the time we reach our mid to late 40s, DHEA levels can be quite low.

DHEA is produced in the adrenal glands early in the morning and declines quickly during the day as it is cleared by the kidneys. The ovaries and the testes secrete small amounts of DHEA. It is unclear what role it can play in cancer. In some cases, it can boost the immune function. In one study it was concluded that DHEA inhibited cell growth and induced apoptosis in BV-2 cells; in addition, the effects were inversely associated with glucose concentration.[54] In another instance, DHEA caused a proliferation of estrogen receptor (ER)-positive breast cancer cells.[55] There still is a great deal more we need to learn about this hormone, which exceeds all other steroid hormones in our body.

DHEA is sold over the counter in various degrees of potency. Because of potential side effects and the way it interplays with other hormones in the body, an individual should be under the supervision of a doctor. Blood tests have to be run to assess current levels and to monitor. DHEA supplementation might be helpful for someone over 50 but I did not find any research identifying its benefits for younger people.

Melatonin

Melatonin is a hormone derived from serotonin, produced by the pineal gland. It regulates the biorhythms of the body and helps in regulating our sleep-wake cycles. It also has antioxidant properties. Recent studies have shown that low levels of melatonin are found in women with breast cancer.[56]

Cortisol

Cortisol secretes from the adrenal glands when the body undergoes stress. Adrenal glands are located on top of each kidney. Cortisol plays a big role in glucose distribution throughout the body. Daily levels are highest when blood glucose levels are lowest. If there are high levels of glucose intake, it can upset the balance with cortisol. When the body produces an over-abundance of cortisol due to long-term stress, it can suppress the immune system and lead to serious illness and possibly cancer.

Chapter 15
Inflammation

Inflammation plays a big role in cancer. Inflammation is associated with the body's immune and endocrine systems' response to tissue damage or irritation, as well as to dietary imbalances, deficiencies, illness and physical injury. An overactive immune system activates an inflammatory reaction, and a weakened immune system opens the door to cancer and other debilitating ailments.[57, 58]

One example is an injury to the head that results in brain inflammation. Internally, several proteins leave the bloodstream and rush to defend and repair tissue damage. Free radicals contribute to inflammation by breaking down healthy cells. These cells become sticky and adhere to other healthy cells, clogging up the system.

Infections trigger an immune response. An estimated 30% of cancers involve inflammation. Abnormal cell division is created by a protein called kappa B (NF-kB). It not only is found in cancer, but also in a multitude of diseases such as Alzheimer's disease, allergies, asthma, autoimmune disease, cardiovascular disease, osteoarthritis, respiratory disease and rheumatoid arthritis.[59]

Short-term inflammation can be a good thing. It helps you heal and generates an immune response to stop infection. When new cells develop, an open wound can heal. Signals to watch out for involve persistent chronic inflammation and swelling, stiffness and pain. This is a clear indication that something is wrong. Patients who are undergoing chemotherapy have major inflammation issues due to the drugs used in treatment. To keep this in check, oncologists routinely prescribe steroids. These play an integral role in helping the body cope with toxic effects.

Chapter 16
Chemo Brain

Chemotherapy drugs used to kill cancer cells may also impair normal brain function. I can attest to that fact. My short-term memory function was not stellar during chemotherapy. I could not retain a phone number for more than three seconds when dialing the telephone. Not remembering I had just taken my medications five minutes before was distressing. In a simple conversation, word retrieval was challenging at times.

For the most part, the oncology community has discounted the concept of "chemo brain" because of the lack of research support. Because of my constant complaints, my good friend Helen, a retired RN, bought a book for me that she found at the UCLA bookstore on this very topic.[60] It was so enlightening to have a name for what I was experiencing and to read first-hand accounts from patients about their issues with it. There also was supportive scientific evidence. The book also addressed ways to alleviate the effects of chemo brain which I followed and have recovered.

Within days of reading the book, an article with the headline "Chemo Brain May Last 5 Years or More" appeared in The New York Times in May of 2011. The findings in the article suggested that the cognitive losses that seem to follow many cancer treatments have shown to be far more pronounced and longer-lasting than commonly believed.[61]

A patient suffering with this condition can do "brain exercises," keeping the brain active. To compensate for memory loss, a patient can make notes and lists. In a study published by Japanese scientists in 2008, concentration and accuracy in voluntary control of hand, shoulder, and leg movements increased by simple gum chewing. The researchers used MRI to reveal that participants had increased signals in the prefrontal cortex when chewing gum with moderate force, most likely due to greater increase in the signal from the brain and increased blood flow. This activated other brain regions including the hippocampus, which is particularly important for memory.[62]

Chapter 17
Radiation

As of 2010, approximately 70 million CT scans were performed annually in the United States. This is a threefold increase since 1993.[63] Rarely do we question our lifetime radiation doses, or for that matter, what a single CT scan radiates. In fact, in a survey conducted in 2007 by the New England Journal of Medicine, physicians were surveyed on how they viewed CT scans in terms of radiation doses as compared to other radiology procedures. The results showed that about 75% of the group significantly underestimated the radiation doses from a CT scan and 53% of radiologists and 91% of emergency room physicians did not believe CT scans increased the lifetime risk of cancer.

This lack of physician awareness translates to a lack of public and patient awareness. Very few people know the radiation dosage of an X-ray versus the radiation received from a CT scan.

X-rays are absorbed in different amounts in the human body depending on density and the organs targeted. An X-ray consists of electromagnetic waves of energy and ionized radiation.

In ionized radiation, there is enough energy exposure to cause stripping from atoms. This breaks chemical bonds of molecules that give matter structure. Too much radiation causes mutations in the body's cells.

A person's radiation exposure and health risk is measured in roentgen of gamma radiation (rem–roentgen equivalent in man) or unit sieverts. One sievert is equal to 100 rem. A smaller unit of measurement used in X-rays and CT scans is the millisievert (mSv), which is one thousandth of a sievert. One chest X-ray amounts to around 0.1 mSv. This affects three cells in one billion. Most bodies can repair this type of cell damage.

The scientific community has established that a 100 mSv annual dose of radiation increases lifetime cancer risk to five in 1000 people. Human exposure to 5,000 mSv at one time can be considered fatal. Humans receive an average natural background dose of radiation up to 3 mSv annually. People who have careers in aviation, medicine, or outdoor sports have higher exposure rates due to receiving additional background radiation than the average person.

A CT scan uses ionized radiation combined with computer technology to produce detailed, cross-sectional images (64 slices) of the area of the body in question. This means many images taken from all angles are combined. A chest CT scan is 8 mSv, which is approximately 400 times that of a chest X-ray. In a study conducted in 2004, though, researchers discovered that even with the same CT settings, different scanners were calibrated to produce different doses of radiation. They estimated a variance of up to 35%.[64]

Physicians in the United States rely on CT scans and other diagnostic imaging procedures to make accurate and speedy diagnoses. Today, people are questioning high radiation dose exposures. Informed physicians and other medical professionals realize that young and middle-aged adults have the potential for over-exposure to radiation during their lifetime and face a higher risk of a secondary cancer. As a result, physicians are limiting CT scans when possible.

Over the past seven years, I received CT scans, X-rays, PET scans, ultrasounds and MRIs. I did have concerns early on in the diagnostic process over my exposure to these tests, but completed them anyway. We needed them prior to surgery and for diagnosing how far my cancers had progressed. However, in 2010, while undergoing treatment for CLL, I researched the radiation exposure of CT scans.

What I found was revealing. It got me thinking about whether it was necessary to have a CT body scan every few months while undergoing chemotherapy. Perhaps some other test would be capable of the same desired results and be less risky and expensive.

I requested to have ultrasounds and MRIs whenever possible because there is no radiation exposure involved in these tests. Ultrasound uses sound waves and MRI employs a magnetic field and radio waves to create an image of the inside of the human body.

Another thought was unless a patient has their medical records from birth of every X-ray or scan performed there is no cumulative data available on a person's lifetime exposure of radiation. Therefore, as individuals, we really do not know how cumulative doses of radiation contribute to cancer or other diseases.

There is a difference between exposure to radiation from the environment (as in inhaled radioactive contamination) versus radiation exposure from a controlled external source such X-ray or CT. Radioactive contamination that is inhaled goes directly into your body; where it lands is anyone's guess.

The late John William Gofman, PhD. was a Professor Emeritus of Molecular and Cell Biology at the University of California at Berkeley. He spent a good part of his career researching the effects of radiation on the human body. In his 1990 book, he stated "By any reasonable standard of biomedical proof, there is no threshold level (no harmless dose) of ionizing radiation with respect to radiation mutagenesis and carcinogenesis"—a conclusion supported in 1995 by a government-funded radiation committee.[65]

In his 1996 book, he provided evidence that medical radiation is a necessary co-actor in about 75% of the recent and current breast cancer cases in the United States.[66] His conclusion from his extensive research was controversial amongst his peers. He estimated that the lifetime cancer mortality risk of a single full-body CT scan was about one in 1,250 people. For a 45-year old adult, it not where to was about one in 1,700.

Lifetime Exposure to Radiation

Unless a patient has their medical records from birth of every X-ray or scan performed there is no cumulative data available on a person's lifetime radiation exposure. Therefore, as individuals, we really do not know how cumulative doses of radiation contribute to cancer or other diseases.

The only long-term study regarding radiation exposure available is of the 86,572 atomic bomb survivors in Hiroshima, Japan. Survivors who received between 5 and 100 mSv of radiation (an average of 29 mSv) had an estimated 5% death rate from cancer. Survivors later died from heart disease, stroke, digestive diseases and respiratory diseases. Other noncancerous diseases that stemmed from radiation exposure were elevated by 14% during the last 30 years of follow-up.[67]

This study has value relative to what an average of 29 mSv can do to the human's body. Researching how these exposures differ would take more investigative work. Exposure can also occur by ingesting radiation through food and water supplies, which can be even more dangerous.

Adolescence is a particular fragile time in life to have radiation exposure. Research has revealed it can lead to cancer later in life. In 2000, a study conducted by the U.S. Scoliosis Cohort took place on the records of 5,573 female patients with scoliosis treated at 14 orthopedic medical centers in the United States between 1912 and 1965. It concluded patients less than 20 years old had many radiograph exposures. Their risk for breast cancer later in life increased significantly and correlated directly with the increase in number of radiograph exposures received for scoliosis during childhood and adolescence.

The fact the study took place during a time when older radiology equipment had been used does not negate the repeated radiation received by young patients during their growth period. In my example, I was diagnosed with scoliosis at the end of my growth period and received very few X-rays. From the beginning, to the end of treatment was six months. It is interesting that studies show that women diagnosed with scoliosis as children are 50% more likely to end up with breast cancer.[68]

In July 2009, a highly controversial article in the Archives of Internal Medicine, a peer-reviewed journal of the AMA, warned that patients who undergo coronary artery calcium screening exams every five years put themselves at risk for developing cancer. Physicists from NIH and Columbia University warned that as many as 42 in every 100,000 of these patients between the ages of 45 and 75 will develop radiation-induced cancer, most likely lung cancer, breast cancer and leukemia. An accompanying editorial noted there was no standard protocol for the quantification of coronary artery calcium scans.

It could be that these tests are doing more harm than good when used repeatedly. Machines though can be programmed incorrectly, malfunction, or involve human technical errors. For example, the FDA and the Los Angeles County Department of Health Services because of some problems investigated a couple of hospitals in Los Angeles.

Cedars-Sinai Medical Center in Los Angeles reported that approximately 260 patients who had CT scans performed between February 2008 and August 2009 received eight times the normal dose of radiation. Cedars-Sinai officials stated the radiation overdoses were due to hospital error. Hospital technicians had changed the default CT settings in February 2008 as part of a new protocol and then failed to reset the machine to the normal dosage settings for approximately 18 months. The error was discovered in August 2009, after some patients who had CT scans reported symptoms of radiation overdose, including hair loss and reddening of the skin.[69]

A second hospital, Glendale Adventist Medical Center in Los Angeles, was discovered to have ten patients who received radiation treatment three to four times the normal dose.[70] In response, the FDA issued an advisory to healthcare professionals to review their CT scan protocols and procedures to prevent future errors. This is not the only facility with this problem and probably not the last.

In 2007, the University Of San Francisco School Of Medicine published a study on the health risks of CT scans. Funded by the National Institute of Biomedical Imaging and Bioengineering along with The National Cancer Institute, they concluded the risk to individuals was likely small, but because of the large number of persons exposed annually, even a small risk could translate into a considerable number of future cancers. For example, the risk of getting cancer in certain groups of patients with certain kinds of scans was as high as 1 in 80. They called for a greater standardization of CT scan radiation for medical safety issues. They found dose variations among machines registering as high as 15%. An additional 5% was added if the machines were not adjusted for children. [71]

Dr. Rebecca Smith-Bindman, a professor in residence in the Department of Radiology at the University of San Francisco (USFS) and her team collected data from 1,119 patients who received 11 common types of CT scans performed at four San Francisco-area hospitals. For each type of CT scan, the dose of radiation varied widely within and across hospitals. There was a 13-fold variation, on average. Because patients come in different sizes, some ability to vary the radiation dose is necessary to produce good diagnostic-quality pictures. The doses discovered and amount of variability were considered excessive. For example, the dose of radiation for a multiphase abdomen-pelvis CT study ranged from 6-90 mSv. The average dose was 31 mSv. Ninety mSv is equivalent to "many thousands of chest X-rays. [72]

Radiation experts recommend we receive less than 1 mSv a year beyond natural background radiation (3 mSv), not counting medical tests. [73] Since we have to do these tests at times, there are many alternatives. Those available are machines such as ultrasound, thermography and MRIs. Any of these options will mitigate radiation exposure.

Should you need to have CT scans or X-rays, check with your physician on possible supplements that can minimize the effects of radiation. There is a wealth of information to support the theory that antioxidants help protect our bodies from free radical formation. The Society of Interventional Radiology reports that a combination of antioxidants consumed prior to a medical imaging study involving radiation could help protect against damaging effects. Vitamin C and glutathione taken orally was found to reduce DNA injury.[74] Other antioxidant nutrients recommended are black and green tea, spirulina, chlorella and kelp, beans and lentils.

Radiation Therapy

As mentioned earlier, excessive radiation exposure can predispose people to cancer. It is ironic we also use it to treat cancer. More than half of all cancer patients receive treatment with radiation. Because of this, I have included information on the technology used to keep you better informed. Certain types of cancers respond well to radiation in terms of reducing the size of tumors and killing cancer cells. Radiation is utilized before or after surgery, or both.

The technology for radiation therapy has developed dramatically over the years. There are computerized machines that can target specific parts of the body, zoom in on a tumor and not affect the tissue around it. Radiation therapy can stop the division of cells. Note that this means all cells, not just cancerous cells.

Gamma knife

Gamma knife is the oldest and most widely used radiation therapy and has been around since 1987. It uses stereotactic radiosurgery (SRS) in which a series of radiation beams converge on a target from various angles. Gamma knife can zero in on a brain tumor without

radiating adjacent tissue. It does this by deploying a high radiation dose at the isocenter of the tumor with a sharp fall-off
in the surrounding tissue. There is no actual knife involved but
a head frame must be employed, unlike cyber knife.[75]

Cyber knife

Cyber knife technology also can treat brain tumors and head
lesions. It deploys real-time X-ray images and uses advanced
image guidance software to track a tumor during radiation
therapy regardless of a physical movement by a patient. Because of the machine's accuracy, fewer sessions are required,
which reduces side effects.

The cyber knife machine can crossfire up to 150 beams at a
targeted tumor from a robotic arm and has unlimited reach to
treat tumors anywhere in the body. With pinpoint accuracy, it
can spare other tissue from unnecessary radiation exposure.

Cases with complications involving lesions that move during respiration require outpatient surgery to implant gold fidu-
cials, which are small markers to guide the robot during treatment to correct for movement.

Tomo therapy

Tomo therapy combines state-of-the art intensity modulated
radiation therapy (IMRT) and SRS with the precision of CT
scanning technology. This groundbreaking technology allows
a single radiation beam to divide into thousands of tiny, nar-
row beamlets delivering radiation from all angles. As the shape
or the location of the tumor changes over time, the angles and

intensity of the beams adjust to improve the effectiveness of the treatment. It can treat the brain, head, or neck, as well as other areas.

Tomo therapy is particularly useful in treating previously radiated areas that can scar and ulcerate. Retreatment is safer and effective for patients who have reached their maximum tolerance from gamma or cyber knife radiation treatments.

Chapter 18
Toxins

We hear more and more today about toxins in our environment and chemicals in our food. I found many studies on how toxins affect the environment, but few long-term controlled studies on the effects of toxins on the human body. If we do not address this problem, are we going to end up with different variations, mutations and shorter life spans? Will the cancer rates in humans and animals continue to grow in numbers? Only time will tell.

Few medical doctors receive training on how to identify toxicities in the human body due to chemical and contaminant exposures. Due to the complexities and long treatment times required, the medical community as a whole is not set-up to address treating patients properly. It takes a specialist to deal with these issues.

There is no real way to know how toxins affect the normal functioning of humans in the short and long term. People can have life threatening and debilitating illnesses from toxic build-up, with little hope of receiving the proper treatment unless they can find a specialist. Toxins can mask themselves into so many diseases.

Mankind is capable of remarkable achievements and I am hopeful we all will work together to clean up the environment, our food supply and products associated with everyday living to ensure a healthy and thriving community. In the meantime, do what you have power over. Make wiser choices in the homes you live in, negate breathing in toxic fumes, smoke and airborne chemicals, watch the food you eat and monitor the products you buy.

Breast Cancer

Breast cancer is a common cancer diagnosed in women today and the second leading cause of cancer death in women. While we continue to race for a cure, 2.4 million women living in the United States have been diagnosed with breast cancer and have gone through treatment. In 2011, an estimated 230,480 new cases of invasive breast cancer, along with an estimated 57,650 additional cases of in situ breast cancer was expected to be diagnosed in American women. Women die every day from this disease.

Breast cancer is a disease touching not only the victims, but also their families and friends. Knowing the possible causes of breast cancer contributes to a path of wellness and helps in the reduction of recurrence of the disease.

Cumulative data and studies conducted by the medical and scientific research communities reveal that one of the most aggressive and disruptive influences contributing to the disease is the excessive amount of hormones found in breast cancer patients.

The culprits, called xenoestrogens, are also called xenohormones. Xeno—refers to something foreign or changed. In the case of women diagnosed with breast cancer, test results are often positive for cancer receptor cells influenced by higher than normal levels of estrogen in women. When it is unopposed by progesterone, it can cause breast cancer.[41] In a woman's body, estrogen has the tendency to promote cell growth responsible for signaling the body to grow blood-rich tissue in the uterus during the first part of the menstrual cycle. It also stimulates eggs in the ovaries to mature. If there is estrogen dominance and not enough progesterone to counter-balance its effect, there is nothing to hold back estrogen from promoting unabated growth.

Why does this happen? Xenoestrogens accumulate in the body over the course of many years because of the body's exposure to a wide variety of chemicals. There are a myriad of chemical reactions in the body that mimic estrogen, which interfere with the body's natural estrogen and cause the liver (which acts as a filtration system) to work harder to excrete estrogen. Why is this bad? Because it influences the cellular DNA and allows bad groups of cells to grow, out of control and travel throughout the body with no exit.

The common sources of xenoestrogens are car exhaust, pesticides, herbicides and fungicides, solvents and adhesives in paint removers, glues and nail polishes, emulsifiers and waxes found in soaps, cosmetics and hair shampoo. Xenoestrogens are also in dry-cleaning chemicals, meat from livestock treated with antibiotics and drugs to plump them up.

In December of 2011, the conclusions of a recent review by the Institute of Medicine (IOM) commissioned by the Susan G. Komen for the Cure organization was revealed to the public. They asked the IOM to look at all existing evidence and the environment to interpret possible causes of breast cancer. A committee was formed to look at all factors not directly inherited through DNA. This covered how a woman grew and developed during her lifetime, what a woman ate and drank, the physical, chemical, and microbial agents she encountered and how much physical activity she engaged in, medical treatments and interventions she underwent, along with social and cultural practices she experienced. This was done to determine whether selected environmental factors were associated with breast cancer and to identify areas of uncertainty.

One of the findings pertains to our topic of toxins. They concluded that since there was a lack of evidence of experimental studies involving humans on environmental exposures involving chemicals, secondhand smoke, breathing auto exhaust, pumping gas or inhaling tobacco smoke, scientists cannot see a clear mechanism for these agents to cause breast cancer. The evidence of risk to humans is still inadequate. However, scientists can see a clear mechanism in animals by which the agents might cause breast cancer. One example is the chemical bisphenol A, or BPA, widely used in plastic containers and food packaging.[76]

Plastics

The plastics we use in our everyday lives—bottles, groceries, health and beauty products, plastic containers and wrappings, all release toxins into our systems. It is almost unavoidable to buy anything not packaged in plastic these days.

There are more than 30 types of plastics used in packaging materials. The common ones are polyethylene, polypropylene, polycarbonates and polyvinyl chlorides. They can be used for strength, transparence, and heat resistance to gases, acidic foods, and as a replacement for glass. Polycarbonates release

BPA, known to mimic female estrogen. Di-2 Ethylhexyl Adipate is a liquid plasticizer added to some plastic food wraps made from polyvinyl chloride (PVC). It migrates into meats and cheeses (fatty foods) when heated.

One way to limit the accumulation of toxins in the body is to take action by reducing or eliminating the use of plastic containers for food storage. I purchase glassware, Corning ware and Pyrex. When heating food in the microwave oven, I use glass containers and remove plastic wrap from frozen foods. I prefer to heat foods in a toaster oven or on the stovetop, which takes more time, but I believe it is worth the benefits. When purchasing foods, I consider the containers and packaging used.

The recycling number on plastic water bottles can tell you which is the safest. The numbers range from #1 to #7, with each number representing a different type of resin. The #1 PET or PETE (polyethylene terephthalate) is common recycled plastic for bottled water and soft drinks and is the safest. Nevertheless, one study in 2003 conducted by Italian researchers found the amount of DEHP in bottled spring water increased after 9 months of storage in a PET bottle. The second safest are #2, #4 and #5. Below is a review of numbers 2-7:

#2 HDPE (high-density polyethylene) products: Milk jugs, toys, liquid detergent bottles and shampoo bottles.

#4 LDPE (low-density polyethylene) products: Cling wrap, grocery bags and sandwich bags.

#5 PP (polypropylene) products: Syrup bottles, yogurt cups/tubs and diapers.

#3, #6 and #7 are the least safe, so try to avoid them. They are used for the following products:

#3 V or PVC (polyvinyl chloride) products: Meat wrap, cooking oil bottles and plumbing pipes.

#6 PS (polystyrene) products: Disposable coffee cups and clam shell take-out containers.

#7 PC or PLA (polycarbonate or polylactide-plastics made from renewable sources) products: Baby bottles, five-gallon water bottles, water cooler bottles, epoxy linings of tin food cans and sport bottles. These release BPA, which is a hormone-disrupting chemical. Do not refill these bottles. Cooling them in the freezer is not advisable. Store all water bottles away from direct sunlight. The shorter the period of time you store them, the better. Drink out of glass containers whenever possible. Buy stainless steel drinking bottles for travel or for the gym. They are safe, recyclable and reusable. Clean them with baking soda and vinegar between washings.

In groundbreaking research, the CDC measured levels of exposure to chemicals by taking blood and urine samples from a group of several thousand Americans in 2005. At the time, there were no regulations in place requiring these tests. The CDC utilized better technology than had been used previously, and discovered there were 148 substances from DDT and other pesticides, metals, PCBs, and plastic ingredients found in the urine of participants. This is astounding to say the least. What is disturbing is that no further scientific studies were conducted on the effects and health impacts of these toxins in the human body. The CDC determined these mean levels, which establish the average poisoning levels detected in the human body for certain chemicals. Why are these common toxins detected in our everyday lives not banned?

Phthalates are molecules that dissolve fragrances, thicken lotions and add flexibility to PVC, vinyl and some intravenous tubes in hospitals. The dashboards of cars are loaded with phthalates and they are in some plastic food wraps. Phthalate molecules can be absorbed into the body through the skin or through ingestion. It takes the body a few minutes to a few hours to dissipate, and levels fluctuate throughout the day.

BPA and phthalates disrupt reproductive development in mice. The National Toxicology Program has raised concerns for potential health issues affecting infants. There are perfluoroalkoxys (PFAs) in nonstick and stain resistant coatings on our pots and pans. In animals, these chemicals damage the liver; affect thyroid hormones, cause birth defects, and perhaps cancer. In both cases, though, the effects on humans are unclear.

Another example of toxic exposure is dioxins. Dioxins escape from paper mills, chemical plants and incinerators. They settle on soil and in water and pass into our food chain. They build up in animal fat and people are exposed to them from eating non-organic meat and dairy products.

Mercury

We have all heard about mercury, which when released from coal-burning power plants, disperses into the atmosphere, falls in rain, washes into lakes, rivers or oceans, and settles on ocean floors. The sea life that feeds from the bottom of the ocean absorbs mercury. Some bacteria transforms into a compound called methyl mercury, which moves up the food chain after plankton absorbs it from the water.

The largest concentrations of methyl mercury settle in large predatory fish such as tuna and swordfish, which we eat along with the mercury and dioxins contained in them. Mining towns in the past released huge amounts of mercury, which swept into lakes, rivers and subsequently dumped into the bays and oceans.

Pollutants

Polybrominated diphenylether (PBDE) flame-retardants are compounds found planet-wide, from polar bears in the Arctic to killer whales in the Pacific. Human breast milk contains it. This compound escapes in the form of dust particles or gases from treated plastics and fabrics. People inhale the dust, and infants crawling on the floor get higher doses of it. Some research suggests these contaminants impair learning, memory and behavior. Impaired reproductive health issues are possible, too.

The reason this is important to us is the ever-growing concern of toxic levels of pollutants in our bodies and the havoc and stress to our immune systems. We have higher rates of cancer now than ever before. Is there a link?

In a study conducted by the EWG published in July of 2005, umbilical cord blood was tested in ten randomly selected newborn babies in hospitals throughout the United States. An astounding 287 contaminants were found, including commercial chemicals, pesticides and pollutants.

In October 2006, a male writer for National Geographic agreed to have extensive blood tests for toxins conducted by Mount Sinai Hospital in New York City. His blood samples were sent to Axys Analytical Services on Vancouver Island, Canada.[7] Axys specializes in subtle chemical detection. They tested for 320 chemicals that could have entered his body via food, drink, in the air and through his skin. It is not surprising that he tested positive for 165 chemicals. Some levels were well above what experts consider acceptable.

Taking all of this into consideration, the best thing for maintaining good health is to try to limit the intake of pollutants and chemicals. Be aware of potential exposures and control the ones you can. I eat organic foods whenever possible, and buy organic soaps, detergents, and cosmetics. I have my hormones checked on a regular basis.

By staying proactive and dedicating my time and money to the things I can control, it feels reassuring and is like an insurance policy for good health.

Pesticides

It comes as no surprise excessive chemical exposure can lead to health risks. In 2009, around 25 million tons of pesticides were used throughout the world.[78] As many as 40% of human cancers may relate to dietary factors caused by pesticides and the interplay between dietary, hereditary and environmental factors.[79] The Environmental Protection Agency (EPA) maintains that exposure to pesticides in both the short and long term have potential health effects in infants, children and adults. These effects range from oral, eye and skin irritation to nervous system damage that can occur within 30-90 days of exposure.

Pesticide research has disclosed that they have the potential to disrupt the genetic components of a cell's genetic code. They also create hormone disruption in the endocrine system, altering the way the body processes its own hormones. The effects of pesticides can result in infertility or birth defects of a fetus exposed during pregnancy.[80]

Pesticides are in our food supply in the United States. According to the United States Department of Agriculture (USDA) Pesticide Data Program's overview of 2008 findings, up to 13 different types of pesticides were detected in food at any given time during testing.[81] The results vary from year to year. No single food uses all available pesticides at one time.

The law allows for pesticide levels as high as 15 parts per million (ppm). Of 11,960 samples of fresh and processed fruit, vegetables, almonds, honey, corn grain and rice samples analyzed, the overall percentage of total residue detections were as low as zero and as high as 3.3% depending on the food.[82] It is important to note that 76.4% of the foods tested in 2008-2010 were grown in the United States. Conventionally grown foods are three to over four times more likely, on average, to contain pesticide residues than organically grown produce.

In California, we import more and more fruits and vegetables from our neighbor, Mexico. Unfortunately, Mexico does not have the regulations we do in the United States. The FDA is only able to sample a small portion of the foods imported from there. It would be interesting to know the pesticide levels in these foods as of 2012. Mexico grows organic fruits and vegetables and companies in the United States, particularly grocery stores, sometimes claim to monitor them.

The EWG ranks foods from the highest to the lowest in terms of pesticides each year. Because pesticide levels vary from year to year, it is important to keep up to date on this information. For example, when tested in 2002, dicloran levels in celery were at 18 ppm. However, in 2008 it dropped down to 1.8 ppm, which was a substantial improvement. In 2010, celery registered the highest levels of pesticides of all vegetables listed by the EWG. Buying organic foods can be expensive, so knowing the foods ranked highest and lowest in pesticides can minimize cost. For a full list go to their web site at www.foodnews.org.

Cosmetics

When we go to the store and purchase health care products, most of us give very little thought to the ingredients. If someone manufactured it, there must have followed the rules to protect our health, right? Wrong. The EWG found that only 28 common cosmetics and toiletries out of 7,500 had all of the ingredients fully tested for safety.

The FDA has no authority to require manufacturers to test their product ingredients for safety. They do not define or regulate the term "organic" as it applies to cosmetics, body care, or personal care products. Companies outside the United States may certify products imported into the United States as organic because they have different manufacturing standards.

A manufacturer can use any ingredient or raw material they want, with the exception of some color additives and other prohibited ingredients. Ingredients in cosmetics and toiletries include 1, 4-dioxane, 1, 2-benzopyrone, lead, ceteareth, polyethylene, triclosan, triclocarban and formaldehyde. To retard microbial spoilage, cosmetics, antiperspirants and deodorants contain synthetic chemical preservatives known as parabens. The ingredients can start with methyl-, ethyl-, benzyl-, propyl-, butyl-, isopropyl- or isobutyl-. Studies have shown parabens have estrogenic activity on estrogen receptor positive (ER+) breast cells, so women or men diagnosed with breast cancer should beware because these chemicals may enter the bloodstream through skin absorption.[83, 84]

Sodium laurel or lauryl sulfate, also known as sodium laureth sulfate (SLS) is found in over 90% of personal care products and is used to break down the skin's moisture barrier. SLS combined with other chemicals may become a nitrosamine, considered a potent carcinogen. Other ingredients containing mineral paraffin oils found in baby oils, tanning lotions or oils, or moisturizing creams could increase skin cancer risk.[85]

Just think about how many chemicals you slather on your body on a daily basis. You get up in the morning and brush your teeth with toothpaste. Then you wash your face with soap. You jump into the shower or bath and use more soap. Deodorant goes under your arms and shaving cream on your face, legs or underarms. Skin lotion is applied. Most women put on probably a minimum of four to five different cosmetics on their faces. To top off everything, perfume or after-shave is applied. Some put on sunscreen if they are going outside. Use these chemicals on a daily basis and multiply by X number of years and it must be staggering the total accumulation of chemicals the body is handling. Remember, these products enter the body through the skin and into the bloodstream.

So, what is the answer? Look for products with ingredients that include as few chemicals as possible. Natural and organic cosmetics and toiletries are not necessarily any safer, though, because they can contain petrochemicals or may only use 10% organic ingredients by weight or volume. If the product says, "Made with organic ingredients," the product must contain at least 70% organic ingredients and can list up to three of the organic ingredients or "food" groups on the principal display panel. Nothing with less than 70% organic ingredients can use the term organic on the display label.

Household Toxins

There is no escaping the toxins in our homes. Our kitchens have phthalates in vinyl flooring and plastics in our food containers, food wraps and utensils. The furniture, blinds, extension cords and electronics in our living rooms have per fluorinated chemicals (PBDD/F). The bedroom also has PBDD/F in the mattress and pillows, carpets, carpet padding, furniture and small electrical appliances. There just is no getting away from them. We live in modern times with modern conveniences. Unless you want to live in a cave, look for products that have lower levels of these harmful chemicals in them. Another option is to find ways to detoxify the body such as infrared sauna, heavy exercise, drinking many fluids, boosting antioxidant levels, maintaining good nutrition and getting adequate sleep.

Chapter 19
Water

Approximately 70% of our planet is covered by water, with 95% of the water in our oceans. Our bodies contain around 70-75% water. I find the correlation between the two very interesting. Water is vital for the survival of our planet and for us. It is not surprising we need to replenish fluid levels in our bodies on a daily basis.

Our bodies lose approximately 8-10 glasses of water per day naturally, so it is important to replace fluids for good health. We lose water through respiration just by breathing. If you live in higher elevations, the loss is even greater because your heart rate increases and your breathing rate is faster.

People generally are not aware they are slightly dehydrated. We usually think of drinking when our mouth becomes dry. Chronic dehydration causes a host of physical problems because the body tries to self-correct this imbalance. It does this by sending water to parts of the body it considers the most important. The brain, which is 85% water, takes priority, for example.[86] Many people drink coffee, tea or beer, which contain dehydrating substances. When we consume these drinks, our body excretes more water than in the drink itself. Warm drinks make us perspire, leading to water loss. Older people tend to be dehydrated and drink less because they lose the desire to drink. As they age, the feeling of thirst diminishes as sensory perceptions slow down. What is the result of dehydration? The cells in our body shrink, losing up to 66% of their water, and the enzyme system within the cell is less efficient.

It makes sense that the human body would have problems functioning well in a dehydrated state. It equates to a battery running at 66% less efficiency. When our energy is low because of dehydration, we tend to eat more food to increase our energy production.

Our blood is about 94% water. A good rule of thumb is to drink 8 to 10 glasses of fluids per day to remain properly hydrated. Water has no calories or fat and is the wisest choice for good health over drinks containing sugar.

Toxic Water

Unfortunately, tap water in the United States was recently found to contain harmful chemicals in 89% of the cities sampled. Chromium-6 is a strong oxidizing agent and is acutely toxic under certain exposure scenarios. It is classified as a known carcinogen in lung cancer, typically when certain workers inhale it through occupational exposure.[87] California EPA scientists have also determined that chromium-6 could be causing cancer by the oral route. These findings are based on an extensive report published by the EWG.[88]

Hexavalent chromium is a metal used in manufacturing steel products, welding, and in production of dyes, pigments and combustion of fossil fuels. Who would have known it also is a component of pesticides used in wood preservatives for outdoor decks and play sets? As the public became aware of the dangers, in 2005, one type of this metal was banned.

In various studies conducted over the past 15 years, chromium-6 was confirmed to enter the body through breathing, eating and drinking. Once it is in the body it converts to chromium-3 and travels through the blood to all parts of the body.[89] This chemical also passes through the stomach unchanged and penetrates tissues and major organs.[90] Chromium-6 was detected in a EWG nationwide study of tap water in 31 of 35 American cities.

In 2009, California officials from the EPA released a public health goal draft that proposed drinking water not exceed 0.06 parts per billion (ppb) of chromium-6 to mitigate the potential for the risk of lifetime cancer for every million people chronically exposed. Even with this proposed percentage, however, officials still are not certain that we will be safe from this chemical. Small children and pregnant women could be at risk as chromium can be transferred to fetuses through the placenta and to infants via breast milk.[91] Of the 25 cities in California whose water was tested, the EWG detected chromium-6 in concentrations from 0.20 to 1.69 in four cities alone. California has a tap water standard of total chromium set at 50 ppb, which is one-half the federal standard. According to these studies, this is much too high. Comparatively, Las Vegas, Nevada had a chromium-6 level of 0.06 ppb and Reno had a level of zero.

One way to make sure your drinking water is free from contaminants is to install an under-counter water filtration system. You can buy freestanding systems that are surprisingly inexpensive. Reverse osmosis is also another way to clear contaminants; some bottled water companies use this process.

Chapter 20
Body Detoxification

We now have established that toxins can play a key role in contributing to health issues. Toxins negatively affect the immune system and general health of individuals, although the effects can be different depending upon the organ or tissue in which the toxins accumulate. Toxins in our diet and environment can cause cumulative free radical destruction. This leads to a biochemical event after many years of exposure and can lead to cancer. Detoxification as a natural bodily function is complex. We do not know whether exposure to a specific chemical will exit the body or become stored.

A diet composed of good, wholesome food choices will support basic detoxification, but detox programs may specifically target the liver, lungs, kidneys, bowels and blood. The liver is a giant filter for the removal of foreign substances and waste from the blood. The kidneys filter waste from the blood into the urine, while the lungs assist in trapping dust and other waste particles as we breathe. It makes good sense to strengthen these organs by reducing the toxic loads they carry.

Glutathione is a naturally occurring antioxidant that neutralizes free radicals. Free radicals steal what they need from our cells and damage our DNA, which can lead to disease and cancer. Glutathione is very important in the functioning of our immune system because it is involved in DNA synthesis and repair. Environmental and chemical pollutants can quickly deplete glutathione levels, reducing our body's ability to detoxify harmful chemicals.

The chemical exposure experienced by World Trade Center rescue workers in New York City in September of 2001 is a prime example of toxic exposure. Emergency workers and residents of New York City had exposure to unprecedented levels of chemicals from burning buildings, which they subsequently inhaled. To this day, the most common complaints are pulmonary and digestive tract inflammatory illnesses.[92] We know that post-traumatic stress and depression also play a part in their overall health, but there is no denying that there have been health and quality of life repercussions.[93]

Many studies support the use of detoxification to reduce the body's burdens of PCBs, PBBs, dioxins, pesticides and drugs. There are many ways to accomplish this goal, and experienced health practitioners know of the methods available. For the purposes of this book, I will cover one effective method.

The far-infrared sauna is one of the best ways to rid toxic chemicals and heavy metals, from the body. Heavy metals have two chemical bonds that stick to fat tissue making them difficult to chelate (remove from the body). Temperatures inside the sauna can reach up to 170 degrees, penetrating two inches deep into the body. Ray lengths between 4-14 microns in the far-infrared spectrum are the safest and most beneficial.

This was one tool used in the Hubbard method for reducing the effects of chemical exposure experienced by New York City rescue workers.[94] More than 500 individuals participated in a *rehabilitation sauna detoxification therapy study*. The results were impressive in that the study revealed a reduction in missed workdays and an improvement in quality of life and family relationships.

If you suspect a need for detoxification, the best way to determine this is to visit a professional with experience. First, some routine blood and urine tests will be taken. Hair analysis sometimes is used to detect heavy metals. Diagnostic tests will determine the levels of toxins or heavy metals in your system. The process of detoxification can take many months or years and can be quite expensive due to not being covered by insurance. There are many environmental detoxification medical centers located in the United States. Private practitioners also can assist in detoxification.

Chapter 21
Acupuncture

Acupuncture is one form of traditional Chinese medicine that originated over 5,000 years ago. The theory behind acupuncture is that the body functions as an energy field known as chi and through 12 major pathways called meridians, which are linked to major organs. Any imbalance in the flow of energy can be corrected by placing needles in specific locations on the skin to stimulate blocked pathways. There are over 1,000 acupoints along the meridians. Health insurance companies generally cover sessions with licensed acupuncturists.

The effects of acupuncture on the immune system are not clear. Numerous studies involving cancer patients failed to clarify whether or not it is beneficial. Positive effects have been proven in adult postoperative surgery to reduce the amount of anesthesia, chemotherapy-induced nausea and vomiting, and for the management of pain.

Pao-Chiang (John) Lu, a licensed acupuncturist who has practiced in Orange County, California for 11 years has an interesting viewpoint. He trained in Taiwan as a medical physician and practiced internal medicine as a doctor there for 20 years. Arriving in the United

States with his family in 1992, he obtained his acupuncture license and has been practicing acupuncture ever since.

While he recognizes western medicine saves lives, he also has witnessed acupuncture being extremely beneficial to cancer patients. John has the ability to see a patient both through the eyes of a physician and an acupuncturist. Patients report that they experience a reduction of pain and fatigue, decreased nausea, improved appetite, decreased anxiety, improved mood and decreased insomnia. He even believes it has helped in improving low platelet counts in some patients.

The one aspect that always concerns him about cancer patients is their interest and ability to keep eating. He believes eating is key in maintaining weight and sustaining life forces throughout chemotherapy and radiation therapies. With acupuncture used as an adjunct to other therapies, improved outcomes are possible.

Chapter 22
Nutrition

Nutrition is as vital to life as the air we breathe. It also is our first line of defense in supporting the body when fighting cancer. If nutritious food is available and affordable, this is the perfect opportunity to change your diet to fight cancer and establish a healthier lifestyle.

A cancer diagnosis is a signal the body is out of balance. The whole body is weak and dysfunctional. As we discussed earlier, the immune system has failed to recognize cancer cells as an enemy and to hold them back. Good nutrition can help strengthen the whole system.

A typical cancer patient has a diet high in fat, low in vegetables and fiber and suffers from malnutrition. Common nutrient deficiencies are good proteins, thiamin, riboflavin, niacin, folate, vitamin K and minerals. It makes sense that if the body is not getting the proper raw nutrients to grow, sustain energy and repair itself; it is going to break down like an old car!

In 2007, the American Institute for Cancer Research (AICR) published one of the most comprehensive reports on diet and cancer ever conducted. The AICR reviewed over half a million scientific studies worldwide and included 7,000 in their final report. An expert panel of 21 world-renowned scientists judged the evidence and developed ten recommendations for cancer prevention.[95]

At the time, the results were groundbreaking, but today we pretty much know what these ten recommendations are because of media coverage and government programs. We hear about staying lean and physically active for at least 30 minutes every day, to avoid sugary drinks and limit the consumption of energy-dense foods such as those with processed sugars and fat. We are told to eat a good variety of vegetables, fruits, whole grains and legumes such as beans. In addition, we should limit the consumption of red meats and avoid processed meats when possible. Alcoholic drinks should be limited to two for men and one for women per day. We should keep the consumption of salt low. Mothers with newborns are encouraged to breastfeed for the first six months and then add other liquids and foods to a baby's diet.

During my cancer treatment, it was highly recommended I seek the advice of a nutritionist experienced with cancer. Fortunately, I found Liliana Partida, CN, who is associated with The Center for New Medicine Clinic in Irvine, California.

Liliana practices what she preaches! She is one of the healthiest people I know and has devoted over 23 years to the health and fitness industry. What I believe sets her apart from others is her direct experience in counseling cancer patients and using nutritional microscopy (used for in preventative medicine) and functional blood chemistry. She uses a scientific approach to nutrition and healing.

I have spoken before about how our blood is the window to our health. This was proven to me by taking a small blood sample via a finger prick, putting it on a glass slide and analyzing it under a dark field microscope. It became quite apparent how "alive" blood really is! We never think of it that way. I saw my own blood cells on a big video screen and watched the movement of cells interacting with one another. The blood sample showed RBC and WBC activity and detected whether there was bacteria, yeast, mold or fungus present. It was amazing to see!

Live blood analysis looks at the condition and quality of RBCs. Healthy RBCs are uniform in shape and size, present themselves as plump circles sitting next to each other, and move around freely. WBCs come in many shapes and sizes.

The results of this test help in assessing the nutritional value of what a person is eating and drinking and can be repeated every 120 days after the RBCs have had a chance to renew. The results are immediate so you do not have to wait a week or two for results.

Liliana's main goal and true reward in working with her patients with cancer is participating in guiding good nutritional choices and creating a strict dietary regimen for recovery. She believes that for self-healing, it is important to stabilize blood sugar, enhance weight loss if necessary, reduce inflammation and plaque and increase immune system function.

At my first visit, we discussed dietary and lifestyle habits. The ultimate goal was to achieve a diet that consisted mostly of 80% alkaline-forming foods such as non-starchy green leafy vegetables and 20% acid-forming foods such as organic meat, fish, eggs, beans and grains.

Clinical research has found a direct correlation to cancer rates and the consumption of meat, cold cuts and milk products, as well as vitamin and mineral deficiencies. The countries with diets rich in vegetables, fish and legumes have proven to have relatively lower cancer rates.

Liliana advises her patients to eat organic foods as much as possible, to avoid partially hydrogenated and trans-fats, and to adopt a low-fat vegetarian diet. She is a proponent of combining certain foods for better digestion and diets rich in vegetables, white meat, fish and fruit in limited amounts. Some of her patients who have strictly followed her diet regime have beaten cancer and remain healthy to this day.

The typical American diet is highly acidic, and even most of our drinking water is acidic. Obesity is often a result of eating or drinking too many acid-forming substances such as alcohol, caffeine, too much protein, fat, vinegar, refined flour products and dairy. Overeating acid-forming foods leaves an acid residue and upsets the pH and natural balance of our body's fluids, blood, tissues, organs and cells. The increase in eating refined simple sugars leeches minerals such as calcium from the bones to neutralize the excess acid waste. This promotes yeast, which wreaks havoc on the body causing health problems. Side effects include fatigue, susceptibility to viruses, and lower immunity.[96] It also increases glucose levels and can lead to disease and cancer. Glucose only gives fuel to cancer.

A healthy human body is slightly alkaline. Alkaline foods are those that have an alkalinizing effect on the body, such as vegetables. Vegetables tend to alkalinize because their sugar structures are complex. Sugars fall into two classifications which are simple and complex. Simple sugars breakdown quickly and cause blood glucose levels to rise sharply. Complex sugars do not affect blood sugar levels so severely. Alkaline diets can also reduce the amount of acidity in the body. All foods can be classified as either acid-forming or alkaline based on their mineral content. Alkaline foods are much wiser choices in safeguarding the body from illness.

People suffering from cancer lack good nutrients because when they eat, the cancer cells consume first and the body receives leftovers. This is especially true in more advanced stages of cancer. Patients can become cachexic, which in Greek means an increase in weight loss and malnutrition. Regaining or stabilizing weight becomes extremely difficult, if not impossible. I can personally speak to this. When I was a Stage IV cancer patient, my daily calorie intake of 2,500-3,000 did not stop my weight and muscle loss. It simply slowed it down. I progressively lost 30 pounds over the course of seven years.

Our Food Production

With the mass production of our food and the soil erosion of fields farmed repeatedly, we have lost some of the mineral and nutrient content in our food. This is seen in double-digit percentage point declines in iron, zinc, calcium, selenium and antioxidants.

In 2000, the United States had 57.3 million acres of fragile, highly erodible cropland that suffered from soil erosion. There was, at the time of the report, 50.5 million acres of land not considered highly erodible, but was later determined to have soil erosion exceeding the total soil-loss rate.[97]

Large corporate farmers in the United States produce most of our food. Conventional farmers use chemical fertilizers to promote plant growth for maximum yield of crops, and use spray insecticides to protect their crops along with herbicides to kill weeds. Organic farmers, on the other hand, yield smaller amounts of crops and use natural fertilizers composed of manure or compost, deploy insects for pest control and plow the land and use mulch to control weeds.[98]

Organic food is more nutritious than conventional foods because of the absence of pesticides. Pesticides disrupt the production of antioxidants in plants we use for food. Plants respond to environmental stress such as insects and weeds. As a result, plants create antioxidant compounds to protect them from attack. These antioxidants in turn protect our bodies when we eat such fruits and vegetables. On the other hand, the pesticides necessary to produce large acres of food become absorbed into our bodies when the food is eaten. Even so, many people believe eating organic food is a waste of money and that there is little additional benefit.

There is some scientific evidence for a greater nutrient content in organic foods. In a study published in the Journal of Agricultural and Food Chemistry in 2004, researchers compared the antioxidant levels of organic and conventionally grown tomatoes. Organic tomatoes had more vitamin C, carotenoids and polyphenols than conventional tomatoes.[99]

In a study conducted on the diets of infants and children in 1993, 23 children aged 3-11 years who were accustomed to eating a conventional diet switched to organic foods during a 15-day study. For the first three days, the children ate conventional foods. For the next five days, they substituted organic equivalents of their usual plant-derived food items. This included fresh produce, juices, processed fruits, vegetables and grain-based products. For the last seven days, they ate their typical conventional diets. Urine samples were collected for analysis in the mornings and evenings throughout this period.

Results showed that the most common insecticides, metabolites of malathion (MDA) and chlorpyrifos (TCPY), dropped when the children were on the organic diet. During both conventional phases of the study, 60% of samples contained MDA and 78% of samples contained TCPY. When the children switched to organic foods, the percentage of samples containing MDA dropped to 22% and the percentage containing TCPY fell to 50%. [100, 101]

Changing your diet can be difficult. I needed the help of my nutritionist for meal preparation planning because I was in a state of shock when advised to change my diet. The information was overwhelming because the foods I commonly ate were the easiest to prepare and of course were the ones that had to go. My entire eating lifestyle had to change.

Change is difficult under normal circumstances and it takes self-discipline. Letting go of fast food, breads, crackers, cookies, sugar, animal proteins containing hormones and antibiotics, saturated fats, cheese and most breakfast cereals with sugar was overwhelming to me. Small amounts of sugar seemed to be in everything I ate.

Sugar was now my enemy. Glucose is necessary for our bodies to function, but in high levels, cancer cells thrive and divide. As discussed earlier, we know cancer cells do not die like normal ones. Cancer cells excrete lactic acid, and the liver (and to some extent the kidneys) converts the lactic acid back into glucose. What do you get? More circulating glucose. [102]

Cancer cells only have 5% of the energy a healthy cell has, so they need glucose. It takes a large amount of glucose to satisfy the energy demands of growing cancer cells. In order to survive and duplicate, cancer cells are like thieves in the night. They steal the glucose supply the body needs to maintain itself.

Sugar decreases the capacity of neutrophils to do their protective job in engulfing bacteria in our blood. Between one to two hours after sugar has been ingested, neutrophil counts decrease rapidly. This condition lasts up to five hours![103]

When I reached the later stages of CLL, my glucose and glycosylated or glycated hemoglobin (A1C) levels (a test that reflects blood glucose levels over a three-month period) were quite high. My physician diagnosed me as borderline diabetic. My diet was good and I was not consuming sugar other than in fruits and good carbohydrates from vegetables. I now know the levels were high because of a high cancer tumor load.

Taking all of this into consideration, what in the world was I going to eat. I had to learn to prepare my meals very simply and, whenever possible, to use organic ingredients.

The normal maintenance diet for healthy people consists of 60% alkaline-forming foods such as green leafy vegetables: kale, lettuce, broccoli, peas, beans, lentils, spices, herbs, seasonings, seeds and nuts. In terms of fruits, those that are dark in color have higher antioxidant levels. The other 40% of a diet for healthy people consists of acid-forming foods such as eggs, fish, meat, beans, nuts or certain grains. When fighting cancer, however, the diet needs adjustment to nourish the body back to health. As such, 80% alkaline-forming foods and 20% acid-forming foods is a good diet.

Oven-baked chicken or fish with added spices, occasional red meat along with steamed vegetables, salads, and plenty of fresh fruit with high antioxidant content (dark fruits) is a good diet for a person fighting cancer. Add oatmeal for breakfast with berries, whole wheat breads, whey protein smoothies, juiced raw vegetables, steamed vegetables or salads, eggs, and limited desserts and snack foods. Snack on nuts or vegetables with dips.

Years after I changed my diet, I now crave wholesome foods and feel like anything else is imitation. I can taste the sugar in sauces in food at restaurants. Desserts are exceptionally sweet.

When I run out of fresh vegetables at home, my body craves them. My taste buds have changed for the better and I do not miss sugar because I feel so much better. My energy levels have increased. I equate it to having a caveman mentality! You just have to go back to the basic food groups.

So, what is the grand prize at the end? Good health—and recovery! It really worked for me. My skin started looking better, and I felt better overall. My immune system began fighting even harder. A back-to-nature type of diet can also be helpful for weight loss in those who are overweight.

Foods that are cancer-fighting due to their antioxidant and chemical properties can be incorporated into your diet. Adding supplements like minerals, enzymes and probiotics were helpful for me, but check with your doctor before using these in combination with any treatment protocol.

Food groups

Below are beneficial food groups for optimal health. If you suffer from certain food allergies, some of these may not be possible for you.

The following cruciform vegetables are best steamed or stir-fried to maintain nutrients: cabbage, brussels sprouts, broccoli, cauliflower and bok choy. The powerful anti-cancer molecules contained within these vegetables are sulforaphanes and indole-3-carbinols. They act as detoxifying agents in certain cancers. [104]

Mushrooms such as reishi, shiitake, maitake, enokidake, cremini, portobello, oyster and thistle oyster stimulate the immune system. Reishi is very powerful and said to be helpful for immune function during chemotherapy. In some patients, it can reduce the side effects of chemotherapy such as nausea, appetite loss and immune system suppression. [105, 106] You can take these in supplemental form as well. Many manufacturers have combinations of these mushroom supplements on the market.

Vegetables such as carrots, yams, squash, pumpkin, tomatoes, beets, and green, red, and yellow peppers all contain vitamin A and lycopene, which can inhibit the growth of cancer cells. Celery and cucumbers are great to use in vegetable juices also.

Onions, shallots, chives and garlic should be your main staples in the kitchen. Add them to everything. The sulfur compounds in these items reduce the carcinogenic effects of nitrosamines found in over-grilled meat and nitrates in deli meats. They promote cell death and regulate blood sugar levels.

Berries are high in ellagic acid and polyphenols (both antioxidants). They can stimulate the elimination of carcinogenic substances. The good berries are blueberries, blackberries, cranberries, raspberries and strawberries.

Citrus fruits such as lemons, grapefruit, oranges and tangerines contain anti-inflammatory flavonoids and are helpful for liver detoxification.

Nuts and seeds such as almonds, walnuts, flax, pumpkin, and sunflower seeds are good sources of protein. Almonds, for instance, contain phytochemicals that have anti-cancer properties. They are also another form of antioxidant.

It is difficult to know what foods are alkalizing and what foods are acidic and I have provided a reference list in the following pages.

Alkalizing Vegetables

Alfalfa

Artichokes

Asparagus

Barley Grass

Beets

Bok Choy

Broccoli

Brussels sprouts

Cabbage

Carrots

Cauliflower

Celery

Chard Greens

Alkalizing Vegetables

Chicory

Chives

Chlorella

Collard Greens

Cucumber

Daikon

Dandelion Root

Eggplant

Fermented Veggies

Garlic

Green Beans

Green Peas

Kale

Kohlradi

Kombu

Alkalizing Vegetables

Lettuce

Leeks

Maitake

Mushrooms

Mustard Greens

Nori

Onions

Parsnips

Peas

Garlic

Green/Red/Yellow Peppers

Pumpkin

Radishes

Reishi

Alkalizing Vegetables

Rutabaga

Scallions

Seaweed

Shallots

Shiitake

Spinach

Spirulina

Sprouts

Sweet Potatoes

Tomatoes

Turnips

Umeboshi

Wakame

Watercress

Alkalizing Fruits

Apples

Apricots

Avocado

Bananas

Blackberries

Cantaloupe

Cherries, sour

Cranberries

Coconut, fresh

Currants

Dates, dried

Figs, dried

Grapes

Alkalizing Fruits

Grapefruit

Guava

Honeydew

Kumquats

Lemons

Limes

Loquats

Mangos

Melons

Nectarines

Oranges

Papayas

Passion fruit

Peaches

Pears

Alkalizing Fruits

Persimmons

Pineapple

Pomegranate

Raisins

Raspberries

Rhubarb

Strawberries

Tangerines

Plums

Watermelon

Alkalizing Proteins

Almonds

Chestnuts

Maple and Rice Syrup

Millet

Alkalizing Sweeteners

Stevia

Tempeh (fermented)

Tofu (fermented)

Whey Protein Powder

Xylitol (stimulates saliva to become alkaline)

Alkalizing Spices

Chili Pepper

Cinnamon

Curry

Ginger

Herbs (all)

Miso

Mustard

Sea Salt

Tamari

Beverages

Beverages are popular and we all enjoy them. Unfortunately, many are full of sugar, corn syrup and other sweeteners. Cancer patients receive no benefit from drinking these due to the obvious additional glucose intake. What is beneficial is juicing vegetables and fruits. Buy a juice machine and find out which combinations of vegetables and fruits you enjoy. You will get immediate nutrition this way.

Supplements

Adding supplements to your protocol while on chemotherapy can be controversial. Some physicians and scientists believe it is beneficial and helps the body overcome the toxic effects of chemotherapy.[107] There is also the belief it detracts from the effectiveness of their protocols.[108] I guess the jury is out on this one. It ends up being a very personal and individual decision and it is advisable to talk with your physicians. In order to determine what supplements you may need, you must take into consideration how therapies affect organ function. Research all the possible consequences of the short-and long-term effects of your particular drug treatments.

For instance, in certain cancers, important minerals and vitamins are depleted. Some chemotherapy drugs can leech important minerals from your body like calcium, magnesium, potassium, and glutathione. Minerals play a vital role in your health. There could be major consequences if these levels drop too low, so supplement use could potentially be beneficial. On the other side of the equation, some supplements could hamper the effectiveness of chemotherapy or cause additional problems.

Some antioxidants are free radical scavengers and can lessen the effects of chemotherapy, and some enzymes could cause problems if certain blood counts are low.

One supplement I found to be helpful for me was a product called Wobenzyme. We all have cancer cells circulating in our bodies from time to time, and it is the immune system that destroys them to keep cancer away. The enzymes in this supplement break down the protein sheath protecting these naughty cells. When exposed, the immune system can recognize and destroy them.

Enzymes are critical in digesting food, particularly in breaking down animal proteins. Trypsin and chymotrypsin are digestive enzymes secreted by the pancreas. When we cook meat above 137 degrees Fahrenheit, the high temperature destroys the enzymes in the meat. Our body has to make up for the loss in the meat by using the same enzymes to help to digest the meat. It leaves little left over for destroying bad cells. Some physicians recommend taking enzymes to replenish this loss.

Spectracell

One test your physician can run to assess the intracellular function of essential micronutrients is called Spectracell. This is a blood test developed at the University of Texas. It can be done in your doctor's office or blood lab and then sent to Spectracell Laboratories.

This test is amazing. It is an easy way to find out what vitamin and mineral deficiencies affect your body negatively, thus affecting immune function. The medical community recognizes how important this is in preventing disease. In fact, most medical insurance companies and Medicare will cover the cost of this test (around $400.00).

Chapter 23
Diagnostic Tests

There are multitudes of tests designed to diagnose and treat cancer, some of which are included in this chapter. Some physicians have their favorites. It is difficult to keep up with the innovations in this field, but I have included some mainstream tests as well as some that are not.

In the United States, patients still have the option to decide what tests they want to have run and to opt out of others. These tests often include biopsies, CT scans, X-rays, MRIs, urinalysis, blood testing, genetic testing and bone marrow testing. The challenge for patients is to decide which tests are best.

Since every cancer is different and unique to each person, there are many tests available to gather information on the make-up and behaviors of specific cancers. This is incredibly important. Every piece of information contributes to the big picture of what is transpiring in the body. If you find value in a test and a physician does not have the facility or desire to run it, find a physician who will. Sometimes it can mean the difference between life and death.

Chemotherapy Assay Tests

Ex-Vivo Analysis – Programmed Cell Death Test (EVA/PCD)

Of all the tests available in treating cancer patients, the one I found the most valuable and potentially life-saving is the EVA/PCD, also known as the Chemo Sensitivity Assay Test. In the lab, live tumor cells from tissue (or blood in the case of leukemia) are exposed to specific drugs. Technicians analyze programmed cell death over a period of one week. In layperson's terms, they look for what drugs one is sensitive to (meaning that the drugs cause tumor cells to die) or are resistant to (meaning tumor cells continue to live even after exposure to the drugs).

An oncologist will use these results to devise a treatment protocol. Some oncologists believe this is an effective test to determine whether a chemotherapy drug will work for a specific patient. Why put a patient through a drug regimen with the hope it will work, rather than knowing it will work? The EVA/PCD test is approximately seven times more clinically effective than drugs inactive in vitro (in the laboratory).

One important fact I want to stress is the test needs to be completed prior to any form of chemotherapy or radiation. The biopsy tissue needs to be fresh and void of exposure from chemotherapy drugs or radiation for best results. This could affect the outcome of the test.

In 2008, I was fortunate to be referred by a friend to Dr. Robert Nagourney, Medical Director at Rational Therapeutics, Inc. in Long Beach, California. He also is an instructor of Pharmacology at the University of California, Irvine School of Medicine and Board-Certified in Internal Medicine, Medical

Oncology and Hematology. I quickly found him to be a brilliant man with the knowledge needed to help formulate a plan for treating my CLL cancer.

Over two separate appointments, we reviewed over six hours of research I accumulated over the span of four years. In addition to our review, the results of my EVA/PCD performed in a laboratory at his office helped formulate a treatment protocol that held the most promise. I later saw Dr. Warren Fong, an oncologist and hematologist in Newport Beach, California in 2010. There I underwent treatment that avoided negative side effects such as infection, bad reactions, nausea, hair loss or loss of appetite. I regained 25 pounds and the cancer tumors melted away quickly.

There are a large number of patient testimonials of survivors living past five years. All were diagnosed with Stage IV cancer and failed other treatment protocols. The EVA/PCD test can be lifesaving. Please keep in mind, there is no test that will 100 percent explain what is transpiring inside the human body. This is because at any given time, we do not know exactly how cancer acts and spreads. There is also no single test revealing how a chemotherapy drug is going to perform in any one person. This test is only as good as the large list of drugs available for testing at the time performed.[109] As a side note, this particular test is presently the most accurate that we have. Progress is still needed in developing new drugs for treating lung, breast, colon and pancreatic cancers more successfully.

One of the reasons chemotherapy does not always work with cancer is because there may be genetic resistance to the drugs. There is no way of knowing beforehand unless genetic testing is done looking for mutations to identify what targeted drugs to use (usually in university hospital settings). A drawback of this is that only a few mutations are revealed in any one test.

There are over 10,000 mutations involved in any one cancer. However, the majority most likely have no significant effect on tumor growth and are not harmful.[110] Typically, there may be up to ten mutations of concern. Even with mutation results, which oncologists routinely test in order to match drugs, tumor cells become resistant to the drugs over time in the same way we experience antibiotic resistance. To make matters worse, some patients do not show mutations for the drugs currently on the market. This is one reason for using the EVA/PCD test. A patient needs as many drug treatment options as possible.

There is no question controversy over this test lingers. The division within the oncology community is in the difference between cell culture drug resistance testing based on cell overgrowth and proliferation as an endpoint and cell culture drug sensitivity testing based on cell death as an endpoint. It really is so simple when you break it down. Do we obtain better results from growing a patient's cancer cells in a tube and seeing what few drugs do not work, or do we have better results from using live cancer cells and exposing them to a large menu of drugs and see which ones kill the cells the fastest and most efficiently? I believe the second option is the most effective.

Some surgeons, pathologists and oncologists are not open-minded about using EVA/PCD. They tend to focus on determining the patient's diagnosis through pathology. Then a cookie cutter treatment protocol is prescribed. This is usually a derivative of clinical trial studies, far from the practice of individualized medicine.

The American Society of Clinical Oncology (ASCO) believes the findings of EVA/PCD are not reliable and they do not endorse it. One of their reasons is there is a long history in the laboratory of live cancer cells not necessarily acting the same in the laboratory (in vitro) as they do in the human body (in vivo). What some do not know is "live" cancer cells plated in 3D micro clusters react the same way as in the human body. This was clearly demonstrated in a study by researchers at Johns Hopkins Engineering Oncology Center in 2010.[111]

The ASCO claims their role is to provide guidance to its members, not to dictate individual practice. Guidelines and technology assessments are not intended to supplant physician judgment.[112] However, they have great influence over the insurance companies that cover procedures and tests, the oncology community and probably universities.

The good news is more leading oncologists and pathologists in mainstream practice are beginning to see the importance of EVA/PCD and are experiencing better patient outcomes. It is no longer enough to simply administer patient treatment protocols that have a statistically slim chance of working and may actually expose the patient to harmful toxins.

There is no average cancer patient and everyone responds to treatment differently. Survival and quality of life issues differ, too. Either a patient will respond to a drug or they will not. To complicate things, cancer cells found in different areas of the body can express different genes and abnormalities. These might need different drugs or treatments conducted separately.

When we take into consideration populations of patients, who have the same malignancy and reveal repeatedly that individuals within the same patient population can have outcomes far from average, there still is a problem in the percentage of successful outcomes. The war on cancer still survives! On average, we keep doing the same things repeatedly and get the same inadequate results.

EVA/PCD can be expensive ($3,500.00 to $4,500.00) depending upon the quantity and complexity of the agents analyzed. Some insurance companies will not cover this cost. If a patient appeals the denial, they may receive partial payment reimbursement.

Perhaps over time insurance companies will change their minds and make these tests standard. Most chemotherapy drugs can be expensive and if a patient fails their first treatment plan, another is tried, which drives up costs, toxicities and wastes precious time. In my opinion, individualizing chemotherapy treatment is well worth the effort and cost to save lives.

Extreme Drug Resistant Assay (EDR)

Surgeons and oncologists are much more likely to use Extreme Drug Resistant (EDR) Assay to detect cell growth. Cancer tumor cells are tested for drug deselection (drugs that do not work) in a laboratory setting with up to five drugs. The goal is to find a drug that stops the growth of cancer cells. If a cancer is aggressive, stopping growth is important. One of the problems with this test is the cells are not tested against a large menu of drugs (say, 20-30) that may or may not necessarily be used for that specific cancer but have the ability to actually kill the cancer cells anyway.

Chemotherapy Resistance Test

ChemoFx

In the ChemoFx test, cancer cells or fluid is removed during surgery or biopsy. Once received by the ChemoFx laboratory, they analyze them. The cancer cells are then grown in their lab where they are treated with a number of chemotherapies specifically recommended for the cancer reported. The test measures both chemo sensitivity and resistance. Their reliance on growing and reproducing cells in tissue is an entirely different procedure than in looking for drugs effective in killing cancer cells. Leukemia and lymphoma are not presently tested.

A three-year study of patients with uterine cancer that concluded in 2009 tested cancerous tissue against five different drugs using ChemoFx. Using this method, findings were consistent with published response rates in studies conducted with the general patient population for those specific drugs. Out of 755 tumor tissues tested, the highest response rate using a two-drug combination was only 66% and the lowest was 23%, respectively.[13]

This study confirms how random drug selection for patients can be. Keep in mind that response rates by no means indicate the patient was cured.

Biopsies

Biopsies involve surgically removing tissue from a cancerous tumor to analyze and stage the cancer as well as to look for gene mutations. Biopsies can spread cancer cells into the blood system, so most patients are advised to start cancer treatment very soon afterward.

Magnetic Resonance Spectroscopy

MR spectroscopy is considered a safe, non-invasive test given by a radiologist that can be used in place of a biopsy. The MR spectroscopy machine has a high magnetic field and shows the chemical makeup of a lump or mass. It can determine whether a breast lump is cancerous because choline compounds, a marker for breast tumors, can be detected with this method. Physicians can also use this method in conjunction with a traditional MRI for breast cancer screening. However, this may not be covered by insurance.[114]

Pathology Reports – Get a second opinion

The pathology report is important in staging cancer and outlines the kind of cancer you have. Generally, the cancer tumor and/or tissue are sent to a lab for analysis after surgery. The results will be a major factor that your oncologist will consider when designing your treatment protocol, along with CT results and blood work.

I cannot emphasize enough the importance of having your cancer tissue analyzed by the best-qualified pathologist familiar with your specific type of cancer. Some pathology departments connected with certain hospitals see a particular kind of cancer throughout the year, such as breast cancer, significantly more than, say, a rare form like testicular cancer. The pathology and staging of the cancer are not always the same across cancers.

Find a pathologist located at a hospital or university facility who has dealt with your specific cancer to consult for a second opinion. Talk to the director of the pathology department where your initial report was generated and sign a release for the tissue slides to be sent to another facility.

Why is this so important? Your treatment plan will be based largely on these results, along with other diagnostic tests. Why not minimize the possibility of having to undergo an unnecessary or harsher form of treatment.

Chapter 24
Tests to Confirm and Monitor Cancer

Before I begin this chapter, I want to reiterate that not all cancer patients benefit equally from the same drug treatment. These statistics may not be very comforting, but 20-75% of standard drug therapy does not benefit patients. Why? Because of a genetic mismatch between the drug for the patient and the disease. We see this with metastatic colon cancer, for instance. Some 40% of patients with metastatic colon cancer do not benefit from standard drug therapy.[115] It is good to make informed choices in selecting tests for your particular cancer. Tests are incredibly important, so do not skip doing those that will be beneficial. Discuss tests with your physician(s).

Anti-Malignin Antibody in Serum (AMAS)

Sam Bogoch, M.D. invented the AMAS test in the 1970s. It detects cancer in your body 1-19 months before it shows up on a standardized test such as an X-ray or other type of scan. It was subsequently patented by Oncolab, Inc. and approved for use by the FDA. It is reported to be 95% accurate on the first test and 99% accurate on repeat analysis. It is not very useful in late malignancy, however, because elevated antibodies no longer are available as evidence of the presence of an antigen.

The AMAS test measures serum levels of an antibody to malign, in which there is a 10,000 Dalton polypeptide found present in most malignant cells regardless of the type of malignancy. A polypeptide is a substance shed from cancer cells. This test has a false positive rate of 5% and a false negative rate of 7%. Other factors can affect the results of this test.

AMAS is a good test to conduct if your doctors are uncertain whether you have cancer. Once you have received cancer treatment and are said to be cured, it is a good diagnostic for monitoring your status. Once the lab has received your blood sample, the turnaround time is 72 hours.

CellSearch

The CellSearch Circulating Tumor Cell Test (CTC) was developed by Veridex and received approval by the FDA in 2004 initially for colorectal cancer. It has since been extended to breast, prostate and testicular cancers as well. This simple blood test detects free-floating cancer cells that can remain in isolation from a tumor for over 20 years (usually in the bone marrow). When CTCs are measured in the blood, they present in only very small numbers.[116]

The number of CTCs is a strong predictor of overall survival and progression of the disease, especially in breast cancer. If the test is performed at the beginning of a treatment protocol as a baseline measurement, it can then be done periodically throughout treatment cycles to determine changes and prognosis.

This is also a good test to have as a baseline in being proactive once cured. If run routinely, action can then be taken to minimize and reduce the tumor load way before it can be recognized in routine blood tests typically used to monitor patients."[17]

Germany has a test called Maintrac that takes the test one-step further by doing a genetic analysis in order to identify the expression of the therapeutic targets and chemo-resistance markers unique to an individual's CTCs.

Firstmark Oncology Health Monitoring Test

In 2010, GenWay Biotech, Inc. launched the "You Test You" cancer assessment test in the United States. They now are expanding their market to European nations. The test is a tool to rule out the likelihood of cancer, and costs approximately $189.00. It enables consumers to be proactive in their health and to conduct a cancer-screening test either at home or through the doctor's office.

This blood test measures biomarkers called tumor fibrin and fibrinogen degradation (tFFDP) by testing properly clotted serum rather than plasma. Serum from incompletely clotted blood may contain fibrinogen, fibrinogen degradation products or plasmid, which is a double-stranded unit of DNA that replicates within a cell independently of the chromosomal DNA fibrin. Higher numbers would indicate the possible presence of cancer or other health problems.

The tFFDP biomarker has been associated with the presence of malignant cancer tumors of different types and is believed to aid in the early detection of cancer. They operate under the true premise that the earlier the cancer is detected, the better off you are. High levels tFFDP are the result of cellular dysfunction. High readings do not only indicate cancer, but can also be the result of other health issues such as clotting disorders, deep vein thrombosis, pulmonary embolism, pre-eclampsia, acute infections, autoimmune disorders, health problems related to smoking, injury or illnesses such as pneumonia or bronchitis, or pregnancy. This is not a conclusive cancer-screening test. You should also use other methods for detecting cancer, especially if it is suspected.

Human Chorionic Gonadotropin (HCG) Urine Test

The HCG urine test was developed over 60 years ago and is extremely accurate, inexpensive and it is not necessary to have a prescription or doctor's orders to conduct it. This test is designed to detect abnormally dividing cells. If cancer is present in the body, this will detect it no matter in which part of the body the cancer originates. Scores of 0-49 are considered normal because healthy people have dividing cells in this range. A score of 50 or higher indicates the presence of cancer requiring treatment. There is an exact procedure required in preparing for this test and the use of certain hormones and steroids must be eliminated prior to providing the sample. It does not work if the patient is pregnant.

The HCG urine test could be useful if you are wondering whether you are on the winning side of ridding yourself of cancer during treatment by using some other method beside chemotherapy and radiation. It could also be used to establish a baseline and progress throughout treatment.

This test is only done at The Nararro Clinic in Manila, Philippines, so your sample must be sent out of the country. The cost of this test is $50.00.

Tests for Lung Cancer

It is estimated that over 200,000 new cases of lung cancer are diagnosed annually. Of those, 150,000 deaths occur. Men and women are equally affected by lung cancer, which usually occurs between the ages of 55 and 65 according to the NIH. Lung cancer is the leading cause of cancer-related deaths in the United States. Approximately 85% of lung cancers are categorized as non–small cell lung cancer, which has traditionally been treated with surgery, radiation, and chemotherapy.[118] Small cell cancer is the second form of lung cancer, usually caused by smoking. Small cell lung cancer is treated the same as non-small cell lung cancer.

Because people who smoke are considered at risk for lung cancer, a test called tNOX is a good test to run if one is a smoker over 50 years of age. tNOX is discussed later in this chapter because it is useful in detecting other forms of cancers as well. People who test positive would then undergo a medical examination and further tests to diagnose lung cancer early, which usually is the key to long term survival.[119]

In 2007, Purdue University researchers conducted a study that examined tNOX levels in 421 volunteers, including people with lung cancer, smokers who had not been diagnosed with lung cancer, and healthy individuals. Among the 104 people with lung cancer, 103 tested positive for tNOX, whereas none of the healthy people tested positive. In smokers over age 40, 12% were positive for the protein that is a possible indicator of early lung cancer.

In addition to tNOX, there are also some new therapies currently in clinical trials for lung cancer, such as photodynamic (light) therapy, vaccines and gene therapy.

Tests for Breast Cancer

The National Breast Cancer Foundation predicts that there will be 200,000 new cases of breast cancer diagnosed in the United States in 2011. This is a troubling statistic, making breast cancer three times more common than other gynecological cancers. In the 1970s, one in ten women was diagnosed with breast cancer. Today, it is one in seven.

Mammogram

Mammograms are the most popular and widely used test for detecting breast cancer. Mammograms use X-rays to locate breast lumps or abnormal tissue by compressing each breast between two plates in the machine. It is unable to distinguish between benign and malignant tumors. The false positive rate ranges from 16.3% for the first test and 9.6% for subsequent tests. When screening begins at age 40, the cumulative probability of a woman receiving at least one false-positive after ten years of annual testing was 61.3% and 41.6% with biennial screening. [120] Another study in 2002 reported a missed detectable cancer rate by mammograms of approximately 30%. [121]

There is controversy regarding the necessity of performing mammograms in women before the age of 40. Arguments against mammography in young women include the fact that their breast tissue is denser and harder to see through. In addition, this would expose women to increased amounts of radiation, possibly leading to cancer over the course of one or two decades. However, there is evidence that mammography can reduce breast cancer mortality in women due when detected in the 50-69 age group. The risk of X-ray induced breast cancer decreases with age.[122]

Nanomagnetic Technology

A new sophisticated technology for detecting breast cancer uses nanomagnetic waves. Nanoparticles are tiny bits of matter that are 100,000 smaller than the thickness of a sheet of paper. Researchers in New Mexico collaborated on pioneering this technology, which has potential advantages over mammography.

In this procedure, nanoparticles of iron oxide are attached to certain antibodies, which are injected into you. The antibody-tagged magnetic nanoparticles fasten themselves to HER-2 receptors on the surface of cancer cells. HER-2, which is a biomarker for breast cancer, is over-expressed about 30% of the time and is found in very aggressive forms of breast cancer.

You are then surrounded with sensitive magnetic coils known as SQUID, creating a magnetic field that causes the magnetized nanoparticles to line up in the same direction. Researchers measure the amount of magnetic decay once the magnetic field is removed. Decay has a linear relationship to the number of tumor-bound nanoparticles, so the number of cancer cells within a tumor can be mathematically determined. They are able to accurately pinpoint 1 million cells at a depth of 4.5 cm. This is about 1,000 times fewer cells than the size at which a tumor can be felt in the breast and 100 times more sensitive than mammography.

This technology has the possibility to detect cancer 2½ years sooner than a mammogram and is able to predict disease progression and monitor the effectiveness of treatment. It probably will be a number of years before it comes to the general marketplace but is good to know it is on the way.[123]

Oncotype DX for Breast Cancer

Oncotype DX is a genetic test that has been used since 2004 with over 135,000 women with breast cancer. Although researchers have determined that only about 5% of breast cancers are a result of an inherited genetic susceptibility.[124] This test can predict the risk of recurrence of breast cancer and identify which patients would benefit from hormone or chemotherapy. If the risk of cancer recurrence is considered low, chemotherapy is not believed to be necessary. The test is appropriate for women who are ER+, lymph node-negative, Stage I breast cancer or Stage II breast cancer. Research shows less than 10% of patients with early-stage ER+, lymph node-negative breast cancer who are treated hormonally receive a benefit from chemotherapy. Of course, outcomes are different for other stages and types of breast cancer.

In Oncotype DX, breast tumor tissue is sent to Genomic Health laboratories where they measure the activity of 21 different genes to classify women as high, low or medium risk for recurrence. Genes control the behavior and activities of all cells. When they behave abnormally, it often is traced back to unusual activity by certain genes. Oncotype DX is a test that can help you and your doctor make a more informed decision about whether or not you would need or benefit from chemotherapy. Over half of diagnosed breast cancers are ER+, meaning that the cancer is fueled by estrogen and has thankfully not spread to the lymph nodes. Studies have shown that chemotherapy is beneficial for only a fraction of people with early-stage (Stage I or II), node-negative, ER+ cancer because only a small number of these early cancers pose a high risk of recurring or spreading outside the breast. This test has been shown to predict ten-year recurrence in patients with ER+, axillary lymph node-negative breast cancer.[125]

Currently, the NCI is using Oncotype DX to identify and assign treatment for more than 10,000 breast cancer patients from 900 sites in the United States, Canada, Ireland and Peru. This is a first-of-its-kind clinical trial called Trial Assigning Individualized Options for Treatment, or TAILORx.

Test results have an average turnaround time of 10-14 days for gene expression. The cost of the test was $4,075.00 in 2010. Most insurance companies (around 95%) will pay for the test.

MammaPrint Assay Test for Breast Cancer

The MammaPrint assay test helps determine the need for lumpectomy versus mastectomy, as well as the need for chemotherapy, hormone therapy or targeted biological therapy. It requires fresh tissues to be collected and stored in a RNA preservative solution. This test analyzes over 70 genes in women under 61 years of age with either ER+ or ER-,lymph node-negative breast cancer. However, this test is only effective in analyzing early-stage breast cancers to ascertain the level of risk for recurrence and possible metastasis.

A research study published in 2010 examined the 70-gene signature in terms of survival in lymph node negative breast cancer.

Women in the study were divided into high and low risk groups based on the 70-gene signature classification and on clinical risk classifications. The researchers also utilized computer software for predicting clinical survival.[126] Low risk patients were those with a five-year distant metastasis-free survival probability greater than 90%. Researchers concluded that the 70-gene signature improved quality-adjusted survival in lymph node negative breast cancer.

Breast Cancer Risk Tests

There are tests available to determine one's lifetime risk of developing breast cancer. These tests are for people who have known mutations, alterations or genetic predispositions to cancer. An example would be cancers that run in families, such as breast or ovarian cancer. The BRCA1 and BRCA2 genes are known markers for breast and ovarian cancers. Cancer in women who have this genetic marker are usually diagnosed at younger ages.

Another study of genetic predispositions to cancer conducted by Yale University and published in July of 2010 concluded that women with the KRAS gene mutation developed ovarian cancer 61% of the time when they also had a family history of breast and ovarian cancer. This typically develops after menopause.[127] Another risk marker for ovarian cancer is hypodentia, which is a condition in which a person is missing six or more teeth because they never developed.[128]

Thermography

Thermography is another name for thermal infrared imaging. A machine takes picture images called thermo grams. These multi-color images show different degrees of heat in unique patterns associated with skin temperature, created by increased or decreased blood flow. Normal areas will show as cool without evidence of suspicious blood vessel activity. Since tumors can generate heat and need a greater blood supply than normal tissue, areas with cancer might appear with an increase in temperature and vascularity (angiogenesis). Each thermo gram uses a numerical scale from Th1-Th5. Th1 is good and means that there are no detectable abnormalities. A score of Th4 or Th5 means that there is a possibility of breast cancer.

The FDA has approved thermography in conjunction with mammograms for the early detection of breast cancer. Thermography can detect activity in the breasts up to 8-10 years earlier 95% of the time, long before a tumor shows on a mammogram. Therefore, thermography is an option before having a mammogram.

The technology for this test has improved over the years and a skilled technician can see disturbances in the body's metabolic processes reflecting areas of inflammation and degeneration. Because thermo grams generate highly specific thermal patterns in each person, a unique "thermal signature" should remain the same over the years. For this reason, it is prudent to have a baseline for annual check-ups.

Because early detection is key to successfully treating breast cancer, this is a good tool for monitoring the breasts. Mammography can result in false negatives, or missing tumors that actually exist. This depends upon location and is more common in early stages of the disease. Statistics show that biopsied tumors detected via mammography are benign 75% of the time. This is a frightening and expensive process to go through, only to find that the tumor is benign.

Another thing to consider is that mammography uses ionizing radiation up to 1,000 times greater than a single chest X-ray. If a premenopausal woman has sensitivity to radiation, she can increase breast cancer risk by 10% for each breast over a ten-year period of time.[129]

Thermography is not covered by insurance and runs between $300.00 and $400.00.

Tumor Marker Tests

Some say our blood is the window of our health. A great deal is determined medically by the state of one's blood, but only a small percentage of cancers can be detected via the blood. Certain cancers such as leukemia, CLL, and CML reveal themselves in the blood by changing the shape and count of WBCs, cause an increase in lymphocytes, and decrease levels of RBCs and hemoglobin. Protein testing can aid in the detection of abnormal immune system proteins called immunoglobulins. When the cancer multiple myeloma is present, immunoglobulins can become elevated.

Tumor marker tests detect chemicals released into the blood, urine or tissues by cancer tumor cells. However, it is also important to note that normal cells in the body might have elevated readings for other reasons and the test results do not necessarily denote cancer. This is why tumor marker tests are not as reliable in diagnosing cancer. Other tests are necessary for proper diagnosis.

Immunoglobulin tests include:

(1) Prostate-specific antigen (PSA) for
prostate cancer,

(2) Human chorionic gonadotropin (HCG) for testicular
cancer and ovarian cancer.

(3) Cancer antigen 125 (CA125) for ovarian cancer,

(4) Alpha-fetoprotein (AFP) for liver cancer.

These tests are done periodically throughout cancer treatment
to monitor how well a patient is responding.

Tests for Prostate Cancer

Prostate cancer is the most common cancer in men and the second leading cause of cancer-related deaths in the United States.

tNOX – Tumor Associated NOX

In September of 2006, researchers identified a protein called tNOX only present in the blood of people with cancer. tNOX is a tumor marker for all cancers and the higher the levels, the worse the disease. A low level of tNOX in an individual with cancer is thought to indicate cancer that is potentially curable.

tNOX is a useful test for prostate cancer because men with high PSA levels do not necessarily have cancer. However, the tNOX enzyme is only present in a blood test if there is cancer. Researchers have determined that in men whose prostate cancer continued to progress based on PSA levels, 60% more tNOX was present in their blood than in men whose disease was stable or whose PSA was falling. tNOX could be extremely useful in other types of cancer, and could be used as part of a panel of markers to detect cancer and monitor its progression.[130]

PSA Test

The PSA blood test is designed to detect PSA that circulates in the blood. PSA is secreted exclusively by prostatic epithelial cells, and its serum concentration is increased in men with prostatic disease, including cancer. This test is widely used as a diagnostic tool.

The PSA test is only 60-70% accurate because PSA is a surrogate marker and not specific to prostate cancer. Other conditions such as inflammation and benign prostatic hyperplasia can also cause serum PSA levels to increase. There is also a high rate of false-positive results in nearly two thirds of the tests performed due to loss of gene function in certain regions.

Men found to have elevated levels of PSA are often referred for a biopsy to check for tumor involvement. Tests that reduce the need for painful biopsies are awaiting approval in the United States.

PROGENSA PCA3 Test

PROGNESA PCA3 is a urine analysis that detects a gene that is highly over-expressed in more than 90% of prostate cancers. This can be quantified in urine specimens following a digital rectal examination. Studies have shown that because PCA3 is highly specific to prostate cancer. It predicts the results of repeat biopsies more accurately than traditional PSA testing.

Physicians may find this test will help in deciding whether patients require aggressive treatment and follow-up or just a watchful wait and see approach. Gen-Probe, Inc. developed this test and released it commercially in Europe in 2006. A clinical trial involving 507 men that previously had negative prostate biopsies in the United States began in August of 2009 and concluded in May of 2010. As of September, 2011 the test is awaiting FDA approval.

GST-P1 and APC Assay Tests

Studies have shown that hyper-methylation of the promoter regions of the Glutathione-S-Transferase (GST-P1) and Adenomatous Polyposis (APC) genes occur at a significantly higher frequency in prostate cancer samples than in benign conditions of the prostate gland. Tests can extract DNA from tissue samples to check for these conditions.

Gene methylation assays may be used as an adjunct to histopathology in patients in whom prostate disease is considered possible. It has been shown that the mutation levels of genes, such as GST-P1, may increase with patient age; therefore, age should be considered along with other clinical factors in the interpretation of test results.

Test for Colon Cancer

Deep-C Trial

This is a new test that can detect tumor-specific alterations or methylations in the DNA of cells shed into stool from cancerous or precancerous lesions. Exact Sciences, a molecular diagnostics company in Wisconsin, have developed it. DNA methylation is a process by which a cell can modify its DNA in order to alter expression of a given gene's product, usually a protein. The test is done at home and involves no diet or medication restrictions or bothersome bowel preparation. This is considered an amazing breakthrough.

A clinical study investigating the potential benefit of this test enrolled 1,100 patients with a median age of 60 at the Mayo Clinic in Rochester, Minnesota. The test detected 64% of precancerous tumors less than a half inch in size and 85% of cancers with tumors on both sides of the colon! What is even more stunning is that 87% of the cancers were Stage I through III, which are considered the most curable and 69% percent were Stage IV, the most advanced. Further clinical trials began in June of 2011 with a much larger patient population of individuals between the ages of 54 and 84 at risk for colorectal cancer. Data from this study will be submitted to the for FDA for premarket approval.[131]

Fecal Occult Blood Test (FOBT)

This is a non-invasive test for early detection of colorectal cancer and for determining cancer stage. The test can detect hidden

blood in stools, as in case of internal bleeding. It is a simple procedure, and physicians have patients perform the test at home.

Dr-70 Immunoassay

Dr-70 is a blood test that detects cancer in the gastrointestinal
tract that has been in use since 1982. This test detects a protein called plasminogen activator (a substance that breaks down
clots) that is present in high levels in malignant cells. The test
has a sensitivity of 91% and a specificity of 93%

Conclusion

This whole journey is an important wakeup call! Now the thing to do is to listen, research, seek multiple professional opinions and talk with cancer survivors. You need to forge ahead and make the important decision to never give up and to seek every possible avenue for the best care and outcomes for yourself. You will find some physicians, depending on the type and severity of your cancer, who will tell you there is no other treatment for your cancer or, in the worst case scenario, say you have only months to live. Find another physician. In many cases, patients who were originally given this prognosis have defied all odds and found other treatments that either cured them or prolonged their lives beyond physicians' expectations.

Other physicians will tell you there is a possibility of a cure or they will do everything in their power to help you fight cancer. Their opinion is never written in stone and likely is based on their experience in treating patients. Patients tend to hang on every word a physician says, but they are not fortunetellers. Physicians can only give advice based on what they know, and some may know more than others may.

Choosing a treatment facility and your physician(s) is a very personal decision. You should ask yourself, "What am I comfortable doing and where am I comfortable doing it?" Some people want to be located close to home for emotional and family support. Some do not mind travelling long distances for treatment. Your emotional happiness is just as important as your physical needs. Miracles happen every day in people who have positive attitudes and who have the self-discipline to adhere to strict protocols of treatment.

No one knows yourself better than you do. It might be difficult at times to get in touch with your feelings, but that is where peace and quiet comes in. Allow yourself the space to explore what you want your outcome to be. Find the strength to control negative thoughts if you have them. One of the reasons almost all studies conducted in human clinical trials give a placebo to patients is because we know the power of the mind and its healing abilities. Your thoughts are as important as your therapy. Being positive and looking toward to the future is a big step toward recovery.

As a patient, you must take responsibility to research the reputation and qualifications of all practitioners and facilities you visit or decide to use. This includes where you go for diagnostic evaluations, testing, surgeries, and treatments, and includes getting a second or third opinion if necessary.

Patients who do their research, have access to qualified practitioners, hospitals, clinical research studies, financial support and insurance coverage for their illness will most likely have the best survival rates.

There are answers out there for your particular ailment along with ongoing medical studies at major universities and cancer centers throughout the world.

Keep safe on your journey. If you are helping someone else, be his or her advocate in a good way. You have gained valuable information by reading this book and can put it to good use. None of us can predict the end result when being treated for cancer; but we certainly can play a large part in the outcome.

It is normal to have good days and bad days during therapy. Try not to let the bad days contribute to negative thoughts about your treatment protocol. The body reacts and then self corrects.

Be courageous in your attempts, stay sharp in your decisions, and keep steady on your feet. Got Cancer? Now What? You know what to do!

Resources

LABORATORY TESTS

Anti-Malignin Antibody in Serum (AMAS)

Oncolab Inc.
36 The Fenway
Boston, MA 02215
800-922-8378
617-536-0850
Fax: 617-536-0657

Email: info@oncolabinc.com

Cellsearch

Veridex, LLC1001 US Highway Route 202
North Raritan, NJ 08869
877-VERIDEX
(877-837-4339) 585-453-3240
Fax: 585-453-3344
http://www.veridex.com/

Ex-Vivo Analysis Programmed Cell Death

Rational Therapeutics
750 E. 29th Street
Long Beach, CA 90806
562.989.6455
800.542.HELP
http://www.rational-t.com/

Firstmark Oncology Health Monitoring Test
GenWay Biotech Inc
6777 Nancy Ridge Drive
San Diego, CA 92121
858-458-0866
Fax: 858-458-0833

http://www.genwaybio.com/

Human Chorionic Gonadotropin Urine Test
Dr. Efren Navarro
Navarro Medical Clinic
3553 Sining Street
Morningside Terrace
Santa Mesa, Manila 1016, Philippines
Calling from U.S.: 011-632-714-7442

http://www.navarromedicalclinic.com/index.php.

Maintrac – Circulating Tumor Cell Test – Germany

Labor und Praxis Dr. med. Ulrich Pachmann
Kurpromenade 2
D-95448 Bayreuth, Germany
Tel +49-921/850 200 (or -201)
Fax +49-921/850 203

http://www.laborpachmann.de

Oncotype Dx

Genomic Health, Inc.101 Galveston Drive
Redwood City, CA 94063
866-ONCOTYPE (866-662-6897)Fax: 650-556-1073
http://www.genomichealth.com/

Spectracell

SpectraCell Laboratories
10401 Town Park Drive
Houston, Texas 77072
800-227-5227
713-621-3101
Fax: 713-621-3234
Email: spec1@spectracell.com
http://www.spectracell.com/

Physicians

Dr. Warren Fong

Medical Oncology and Hematology
361 Hospital Road, Suite 530
Newport Beach, CA 92663
949-574-1610

Dr. Leigh Erin Connealy

Primary Care
Center for New Medicine
6 Hughes, Suite 100
Irvine, CA 92618
949-680-1880
http://www.cfnmedicine.com/

Dr. Robert Nagourney

Rational Therapeutics, Inc.
Oncologist
750 E. 29th Street,
Long Beach, CA 90806
562-989-6455
800-542-HELP
http://www.rational-t.com/

Nutritionist
Liliana Partida

Nutritionist, CN
Center for New Medicine
6 Hughes, Suite 100
Irvine, CA 92618
949-680-1880
www.cfnmedicine.com

Organizations Aiding Cancer Patients

Web sites:

http://www.cleaningforareason.org

Offers free professional housecleaning and maid services to improve the lives of women undergoing treatment for cancer. They provide free housecleaning once per month for 4 months while a woman is in treatment, allowing her to focus on her health while they focus on her home.

http://www.joyfulfoundation.org

Supply handmade lap blankets to hospitals, cancer centers and individuals while receiving long-term medical treatments, chemotherapy, or renal dialysis, as well as victims of spousal abuse and their children. The blankets are meant to be a source of warmth and comfort for patients during long treatment sessions.

http://www.heavenlyhats.com

Collects and distributes new hats of all kinds to heroes of all ages who lose their hair due to cancer treatments or other medical conditions. They want to help every patient in need of headwear for warmth, comfort, courage and strength and will ship the hats directly to individuals.

Web Sites of Interest

http://www.foodnews.org/

http://www.cosmeticdatabase.org/

http://www.allnaturalcosmetics.com

http://www.aquasana.com

http://www.drinkorgain.com

http://www.ewg.org/skindeep.

http://www.gotcancernowwhat.com/

http://www.worldcat.org

http://www.pubmed.com

http://www.jointcommission.org

Bibliography

1.   Bennett, M.P., The effect of mirthful laughter on stress and natural killer cell cytotoxicty, 1997.
2.   Czyzewski, A., Breast cancer patients suffer long lasting-radiotherapy complications. CANCER 18 September 2007.
3.   Ravotuo,Virginia, Radiation: Radiation and the Heart.2011; Available from: http://www.clubreduva.com/community/ask the expert 1/may-2011-spotlight.
4.   Mukherjee, S., The Emperor of All Maladies: A Biography of Cancer Aug 9, 2011, New York: Scribner A Division of Simon & Schuster, Inc. 573.
5.   Levinson, D.R., Adverse Events in Hospitals: National Incidence Among Medicare Beneficiaries, D.O.H.A.H.S.O.O.I.General, Editor November, 2010, Department of Health and Human Services. p. 81.
6.   Goodman, J.C., P. Villarreal, and B. Jones, The social cost of adverse medical events, and what we can do about it. Health Affairs, 2011. 30(4): p. 590-595.
7.   Davis,-D.L., The Secret History of the War on Cancer,2007, New-York: BasicBooks.
8.   Brooke,J.Doran,E.,Verdicts, Settlements and Statistical Analysis 5,8, in Jury Verdict Research,2005.
9.   Koepke,Phd,D.,Pickens-Phd,Gary, Hospitals Continue Financial Recovery, in Research Paper,2009, Center for Healthcare Improvement.
10. Gengler,A., Fight Your Insurer's Claim Denial, in Money-Sept.2011, Money.
11. Tomlinson,I.,P.Sasieni, and W. Bodmer, How Many Mutations in a Cancer? The American Journal of Pathology, 2002. 160(3): p. 755-758.

12. Reuters, T., Cancer Costs to Rise to $158-Billion-in-2020,2011, Fox-News.com.

13. Reichrath, J., M. Friedrich, and W. Tilgen. Vitamin D analogs in cancer prevention and therapy. Berlin; New York: Springer.

14. Simonton, O.C., R.M. Henson, and B. Hampton, The Healing Journey-1992, New York: Bantam Books.

15. Carnegie Library of Pittsburgh, S. and D. Technology, The Handy Science Answer Book,1994, Detroit: Visible Ink Press.

16. Consortium,. ICGC releases new genomic data on cancer ahead of schedule.2011 [cited-October 29,2011];Available from: http://www.icgc.org/icgc/media.

17. Jetter, A., Special Report: Strong Medicine Is the FDA, America's consumer watchdog, understaffed, overburdened,ethically challenged,or merely misunderstood? The Reader's Digest.2008, The Reader's Digest Association:Pleasantville, N.Y., etc. p. 118.

18. National Cancer Institute,U.S.-N.I.O.H.,Office of Cancer Complementary and Alternative Medicine, U.S.N.I.O.H.National-Cancer-Institute,Editor-2011, http://www.cancer.gov/cam/camatnci.html.

19. National Cancer Policy Board, I.O.M., Sources of Cancer Research Funding in the United States. June 1999.

20. Institute, U.S.I.O.H.N.C. Cancer CAM Clinical Trials. 2011 [cited 2011 September 10, 2011]; Available from: http://www.cancer.gov/cam/clinicaltrials_list.html.

21. Huang,H.Y.,et al., Multivitamin/mineral supplements and prevention of chronic disease 2006, Rockville, MD: Agency for Healthcare Research and Quality.

22. Ornish,D., et al., Intensive Lifestyle Changes May Affect the Progression of Prostate Cancer. The Journal of Urology, 2005. 174(3): p. 1065-1070.

23. Kohler, B.A., et al., Annual Report to the Nation on the Status of Cancer, 1975-2007, Featuring Tumors of the Brain and Other Nervous System. Journal of the National Cancer Institute, 2011. 103(9): p. 714-736.

24. Prevention, C.F.D.C.A., The Annual Report to the Nation on the Status of Cancer, 1975-2007 found continued declines in many cancer rates., C.F.D.C.A. Prevention, Editor 2011: Atlanta, GA 30333.

25. Verdecchia, A., et al., Recent cancer survival in Europe: a 2000-02 period analysis of EUROCARE-4 data. The Lancet Oncology, 2007. 8(9): p. 784-96.

26. Smith,N.F.,I Spy:Designer Breast Cancer Drugs. More, August.15, 2011(August 2011): p. 3.

27. Gazdar, A.F., Personalized Medicine and Inhibition of EGFR Signaling in Lung Cancer. New England Journal of Medicine, 2009. 361(10): p. 1018-1020.

28. Winslow, R., Major Shift in War on Cancer, The Wall Street Journal-2011, Dow Jones a News Company: Chicago. p. Front, A2.

29. Alschuler,LisaN.,Gazella,Karolyn A Excerpt from Alternative Medicine Magazine's Definitive Guide to Cancer: An Integrative Approach to Prevention, Treatment, and Healing. Townsend Letter, 2007. 289/290: p. 132-135.

30. Naing A, S.S., Frenkel M, Chandhasin C, Hong DS, Lei X, Falchook G, Wheler J.J Fu, S. Kurzrock., Prevalence of complementary medicine use in a phase 1 clinical trials program: The MD Anderson Cancer Center Experience., 2011, American Cancer Society.

31. Fouladbakhsh JM, S.M., Given BA, Given CW., Source, and M.S.U.I.E.L. College of Nursing, USA. judif129@ comcast.ne:Predictors of use of complementary and alternative therapies among patients with cancer., College of Nursing, Michigan State University in East Lansing, USA. 2005 Oncology Nurse Forum. 2005 Nov 3;. p. 1115-22

32. Parker, S., The Human Body Book,2007, London; Melbourne.
33. Dzugan,S.andA.Scipione,Progesterone Misconceptions, in Life Extension,2006, LE-Publications,Inc.: Fort Lauderdale, Florida 33309.
34. Lee, J.R., J. Hanley, and V. Hopkins, What Your Doctor May Not Tell You About Premenopause : Balance Your Hormones and Your Life From Thirty to Fifty-1999, New York: Warner Books.
35. Prins,G.S.,et.al.,The role of estrogens in normal and abnormal development of the prostate gland. Annals of the New York Academy of Sciences, 2006. 1089: p. 1-13.
36. Lau, K.-M. Estrogen and Antiestrogen Actions on Human Prostate Cancer: A Dissertation. 1970; Available from: http://escholarship.umassmed.edu/gsbs_diss/37.
37. Morgentaler,A., C.O. Bruning, and W.C. DeWolf, Occult Prostate Cancer in Men With Low Serum Testosterone Levels. JAMA: The Journal of the American Medical Association, 1996. 276(23): p. 1904-1906.
38. Biro,F.M., et al., Pubertal assessment method and baseline characteristics in a mixed longitudinal study of girls. Pediatrics Pediatrics, 2010. 126(3): p. e583-e590.
39. Council, N.R.D. Smarter Living: Health Reports-Saving Antibiotics
    What You Need to Know About Antibiotics Abuse on Farms. May 25,2011;Available-from: http://www.nrdc.org/living/healthreports/keep-antibiotics-working.asp.
40. Lee,R.J.M.,J.M.Hanley, and V. Hopkins, What Your Doctor May Not Tell You About Premenopause-1999, New York: Warner Books. 382.
41. Lee,J.R.,D.Zava,and-V.Hopkins,WhatYour Doctor May Not Tell You About Breast Cancer : How hormone balance can help save your life-2002, New York, NY: Warner Books.

42. Morra, M.E. and E. Potts, Choices. A Harper-Resource book-2003, New York: HarperCollins.

43. Writing Group for the Womens Health Initiative, I., Risks and Benefits of Estrogen Plus Progestin in Healthy Post-menopausal Women:Principal Results From the Women's Health Initiative Randomized Controlled Trial. Obstetrical & gynecological survey., 2002. 57: p. 750-751.

44. Administration,F.D. Safety information by drug class. 2010; Available from: http://FDA.gov/drugs/drug safety/informationbydrugclass/ucm168838.htm.

45. Fallon,W.,The Unscientific Bioidentical Hormone Debate, in Life Extension 2009, LE Publications, Inc.: Fort Lauderdale, Florida 33309.

46. Foundation,L.e.,Bioidentical Hormones: Why are they still controversial?, Life-Extension Magazine-2009, LE Publications, Inc.: Fort Lauderdale, Florida 33309.

47. Campagnoli, C., et al., Progestins and progesterone in hormone replacement therapy and the risk of breast cancer. The Journal of Steroid Biochemistry and Molecular Biology., 2005. 96(2): p. 95-108.

48. Herman Giddens,M.E.,et al., Secondary sexual characteristics and menses in young girls seen in office practice: a study from the Pediatric Research in Office Settings Network. Pediatrics, 1997. 99(4): p. 505-12.

49. Cowan,L.D.,et.al.,Breast cancer incidence in women with a history of progesterone deficiency.American Journal of Epidemiology, 1981. 114(2): p. 209-17.

50. Jones, T.H., Testosterone Deficiency in Men 2008, Oxford; New York: Oxford University Press.

51. Travison, T.G., et al., A Population Level Decline in Serum Testosterone Levels in American Men. Journal of Clinical Endocrinology & Metabolism, 2007. 92(1): p. 196-202.

52. Vergel,N.and R. Program for Wellness, Testosterone: A Man's Guide Practical Tips for Boosting Sexual, Physical, and Mental Vitality 2010, Houston: Milestones.

53. Fallon, W., Startling Low Testosterone Blood Levels in Male Life Extension Members, in Life Extension-June 2010, LE Publications, Inc. p. 85-90.

54. Yang, N.-C., et al., DHEA inhibits cell growth and induces apoptosis in BV-2 cells and the effects are inversely associated with glucose concentration in the medium. The Journal of Steroid Biochemistry and Molecular Biology, 2000. 75(2-3): p. 159-166.

55. Calhoun,K.E.,et.al., Dehydroepiandrosterone sulfate causes proliferation of estrogen receptor positive breast cancer cells despite treatment with fulvestrant. Archives of Surgery (Chicago, Ill. : 1960), 2003. 138(8): p. 879-83.

56. Baldwin,W.S.and-J.C.Barrett, Melatonin: receptor mediated events that may affect breast and other steroid hormone dependent cancers. Molecular carcinogenesis, 1998. 21(3): p. 149-55.

57. Challem, J., The Inflammation Syndrome:Your Nutritional Plan for great health, weight loss, and pain free living,2010, Hoboken, N.J.: John Wiley & Sons.

58. Walford, R.L., The Immunologic Theory of Aging-1969, København: Munksgaard.

59. Probst-Hensch, N.M., Chronic age related diseases share risk factors:do they share pathophysiological mechanisms and why does that matter? Swiss Medical Weekly, 2010. 140.

60. Silverman,D.and I.Davidson, Your Brain After Chemo : A Practical Guide to Lifting the Fog and Getting Back Your Focus 2009, Cambridge, MA: Da Capo Lifelong.

61. Parker-Pope, T., Chemo Brain May Last 5 Years or More, in The New York Times 2011, The New York Times: New York.

62. Onozuka, M., et al., Mapping Brain Region Activity during Chewing: A Functional Magnetic Resonance Imaging Study. Journal of Dental Research, 2002. 81(11): p. 743-746.

63. Brenner, D.J. and E.J. Hall, Computed Tomorgraphy An Increasing Source of Radiation Exposure. New England Journal of Medicine, 2007. 357:2277-2284(24).

64. Brenner, D.J. and C.D. Ellston, Estimated Radiation Risks Potentially Associated with Full Body CT Screening. Radiology, 2004: p. 738.

65. Gofman, J.W., Radiation induced cancer from low dose exposure:An independent Analysis 1990,San Francisco, Calif.:Committee for Nuclear Responsibility.

66. Gofman,J.W.and E. O'Connor, Preventing breast cancer : The story of a major, proven, preventable cause of this disease-1996, San Francisco, Calif., U.S.A.: C.N.R. Book Division, Committee for Nuclear Responsibility, Inc.

67. Preston, D.L., et al., Solid cancer and noncancer disease mortality 1950-1997, in Studies of mortality of atomic bomb survivors2003. p. 381-407.

68. Doody,M.M.,et.al.,Breast cancer mortality after diagnostic radiography: findings from the U.S. Scoliosis Cohort Study. Spine, 2000. 25(16): p. 2052-63.

69. Zarembo, A., Cedars-Sinai investigated for significant radiation overdoses of 206 patients,in Los Angeles Times October 10, 2009, Los Angeles Times: Los Angeles.

70. Zarembo, A., Radiation overdoses found at second hospital, in Los Angeles Times,November 21, 2009, Los Angeles Times: Los Angeles.

71. Berrington de Gonzalez, A., et al., Projected Cancer Risks From Computed Tomographic Scans Performed in the United States in 2007. Arch Intern Med, 2009. 169(22): p. 2071-2077.

72. Smith-Bindman, R., et al., Radiation dose associated with common computed tomography examinations and the associated lifetime attributable risk of cancer. Archives of internal medicine, 2009. 169(22): p. 2078-86.

73. American, S., Exposed Medical imaging delivers big doses of radiation. Scientific American, May 2011(May 2011).

74. Staff,L.E.M.,In the News: Antioxidants May Protect te Body fron CT Radiation. Life Extension Magazine, 2011(July 2011).

75. S. Christopher Hoffelt, M. Gamma Knife vs. CyberKnife. September/October-2006;Available from: http://www.swmedicalcenter.org/documents/Cyberknife/OncologyIssuesVol21No5.pdf.

76. Academies,S.I.O.M.O.T.N.,Breast Cancer and the Environment A Life Course Approach. Institute of Medicine of the National Academies, 2011: p. 4.

77. Duncan, D.E., The Pollution Within in National Geographic. 2006, National Geographic Society:[Washington, D.C.]. p. 116.

78. Tadeo, J.L., Analysis of pesticides in food and environmental samples-2008, Boca Raton: CRC Press.

79. Ferguson, L.R., Natural and man-made mutagens and carcinogens in the human diet. Mutation research, 1999. 443(1-2): p. 1-2.

80. Agency, E.P., Pesticides: Topical & Chemical Fact Sheets. 2007.

81. United States. Agency for Toxic, S. USDA – AMS Pesticide Data Program Overview-of 2008 Findings 2008;Available-from: http://www.ams.usda.gov/AMSv1.0/getfile?dDocName=stelprdc5084847.

82. United States. Agency for Toxic, S.-D.o.A. Pesticide Data
     Program-Progress Report 2008-2010. March, 2010;
     Available-from: http://www.ams.usda.gov/AMSv1.0/getfil
     e?dDocName=STELDEV3002094.

83. Beckley-Kartey, S.A., S.A. Hotchkiss, and M. Capel, Com-
     parative in vitro skin absorption and metabolism of couma-
     rin (1,2-benzopyrone) in human, rat, and mouse. Toxicology
     and applied pharmacology, 1997. 145(1): p. 34-42.

84. Okubo,T.,et.al.,ER-dependent estrogenic activity of para-
     bens assessed by proliferation of human breast cancer
     MCF-7 cells and expression of ERalpha and PR. Food and
     Chemical Toxicology : An International Journal published
     for the British Industrial Biological Research Association,
     2001. 39(12): p. 1225-32.

85. Lu,Y.P.,et al.,Tumorigenic effect of some commonly used
     moisturizing creams when applied topically to UVB pretreat-
     ed high-risk mice. J. Invest. Dermatol. Journal of Investiga-
     tive Dermatology, 2009. 129(2): p. 468-475.

86. Batmanghelidj, F., Water : for Health, for Healing, for Life
     : You're not sick, you're thirsty!2003, New York: Warner
     Books.

87. Humans,B, Chromium, nickel and welding. IARC mono-
     graphs on the evaluation of carcinogenic risks to humans /
     World Health Organization, International Agency for Re-
     search on Cancer, 1990. 49: p. 1-648.

88. Sutton,R.and G. Environmental Working. Chromium-6 in-
     U.S.-tapwater-.2010;Available-from: http://static.ewg.org/
     reports/2010/chrome6/chrome6 report 2.pdf.

89. Syracuse Research, C., et al. Toxicological profile for
     chromium.1993;Available from: http://catalog.hathitrust.
     org/api/volumes/oclc/29180923.html.

90. Costa,M., Toxicity and carcinogenicity of Cr(VI) in animal models and humans. Critical reviews in toxicology, 1997. 27(5): p. 431-42.

91. Assessment, O.O.E.H.H. and P.A.E.T. Branch, Public Health Goal forHexavalent Chromium-in Drinking Water August 2009, Office of Environmental Health Hazard Assessment-California. p. 149.

92. Lin,S.,et.al.,Upper-Respiratory Symptoms and Other Health Effects among Residents Living Near the World Trade Center Site after September 11, 2001.American Journal of Epidemiology, 2005. 162(6): p. 499-507.

93. Wisnivesky, J.P., et al., Persistence of multiple illnesses in World Trade Center rescue and recovery workers: a cohort study. The Lancet, 2011. 378(9794): p. 888-897.

94. Cecchini,M.A.,et.al.,Chemical Exposures at the World Trade Center:Use of the Hubbard Sauna Detoxification Regimen to Improve the Health Status of New York City Rescue Workers Exposed to Toxicants. Townsend Letter For Doctors and Patients, 2006(273): p. 58-65.

95. World Cancer Research, F. and R. American Institute for Cancer, Food, nutrition, physical activity, and the prevention of cancer:a global perspective 2007,Washington,DC: WCRF/AICR.

96. Varona, V., Nature's Cancer-Fighting Foods: Prevent and Reverse the most common forms of cancer using the proven power of great food and easy recipes,2001, Paramus, NJ: Reward Books.

97. Toy, T.J., G.R. Foster, and K.G. Renard, Soil erosion : processes, prediction,measurement,and,control 2002, New York: John Wiley & Sons.

98. Staff, M.C. Organic foods: Are they safer? More nutritious? December 18, 2010.

99. Caris-Veyrat, C., et al., Influence of organic versus conventional agricultural practice on the antioxidant microconstituent content of tomatoes and derived purees; consequences on antioxidant plasma status in humans. Journal of Agricultural and Food Chemistry, 2004. 52(21): p. 6503-9.

100. Barrett,J.R.,OP Pesticides in Children's Bodies: The Effects of a Conventional versus Organic Diet. Environmenta Health Perspectives, 2006. 114(2): p. A112.

101. Curl,C.L.,R.A.Fenske,andK.Elgethun, Organophosphorus Pesticide Exposure of Urban and Suburban Preschool Children with Organic and Conventional Diets. Environmental Health Perspectives, 2003. 111(3): p. 377-382.

102. John,A.P., Dysfunctional mitochondria, not oxygen insufficiency, cause cancer cells to produce inordinate amounts of lactic acid: the impact of this on the treatment of cancer. Medical hypotheses, 2001. 57(4): p. 429-431.

103. Sanchez, A., et al., Role of sugars in human neutrophilic phagocytosis. The American Journal of Clinical Nutrition, 1973. 26(11): p. 1180-1184.

104. Pappa, G. Mechanisms of cell cycle arrest and apoptosis induction by sulforaphane and compinatorial effects of-sulforaphane and 3,3' Diindolylmethane on cancer cell growth inhibition.2007;Available from: http://deposit.dnb.de/cgi-bin/dokserv?idn=987648497.

105. Weng, C.J. and G.C. Yen, The in vitro and in vivo experimental evidences disclose the chemopreventive effects of Ganoderma lucidum on cancer invasion and metastasis. Clin. Exp. Metastasis Clinical and Experimental Metastasis, 2010. 27(5): p. 361-369.

106. Kim,K.C.,et.al.,Enhancement of radiation response with combined Ganoderma lucidum and Duchesnea chrysantha extracts in human leukemia HL-60 cells. International journal of molecular medicine, 2008. 21(4): p. 489-98.

107. Drisko, J.A., J. Chapman, and V.J. Hunter,The use of antioxidant therapies during chemotherapy. Gynecologic Oncology, 2003. 88: p. 434-439.

108. D'Andrea,G.M.,Use of antioxidants during chemotherapy and radiotherapy should be avoided.CA: a cancer journal for clinicians, 2005. 55(5).

109. Moss,R.W.,Customized Cancer Treatment 2010,Lemont, PA:Equinox Press. 266.

110. Tomlinson,I.,P.Sasieni, and W. Bodmer, How Many Mutations in a Cancer? Am J Pathol, 2002. 160(3): p. 755-758.

111. Spiro,M.,Cells studied in 3D may reveal novel cancer targets, in John Hopkins University Engineering in Oncology CenterOctober, 2010, John Hopkins Engineering in Oncology Center: http://psoc.inbt.jhu.edu/2010/10/14/ cells studied in 3d may reveal novel cancer targets/.

112. Schrag,D.,et.al.,Correspondence In Reply:Dr. Nagourney: Chemosensitivity and Resistance Assays: A Systematic Review? Journal of Clinical Oncology,©2005-American-Society of Clinical Oncology.,2005. 23(No.15 (May 20), 2005): p. 3646-3648.

113. Huh,W.K., et al., Consistency of In Vitro Chemoresponse Assay Results and Population Clinical Response Rates Among Women With Endometrial Carcinoma.International-al Journal of Gynecological Cancer,2011.21(3):p.494-499 10.1097/IGC.0b013e31820c4cb5.

114. Bartella,L.,et.al.,Proton-MR spectroscopy with choline peak as malignancy marker improves positive predictive value for breast cancer diagnosis: preliminary study. Radiology, 2006. 239(3): p. 686-92.

115. Mamula,K.B.,Precision Therapeutics Inc. prepares to bring new products to market in Pittsburgh Business Times-August 26, 2011: Pittsburgh.

116. Pachmann,K.,et.al.,Chemosensitivity-Testing-of Circulating Epithelial Cells (CETC) in Breast Cancer Patients and Correlation to Clinical Outcome. Cancer research, 2009. 69(24): p. 2044.

117. Nemeroff, S., ND, Circulating Tumor Cell Assays: A Major Advance in Cancer Treatment. Life Extension Magazine, April 2010(April, 2010).

118. Moran, C., Importance of Molecular Features of Non–Small Cell Lung Cancer for Choice of Treatment. The American Journal of Pathology, 2011. 178(5): p. 1940-1948.

119. Barrow, K. New Blood tet May Detect Cancer Early. 2007-December5,2011;Available from: www.healthvideo.con/article.php?id=183&category=Ovarian.

120. Hubbard,R.A.,etal.,Cumulative Probability of FalsePositive Recall or Biopsy Recommendation After 10 Years of Screening Mammography. Annals of Internal Medicine, 2011. 155(8): p. 481-492.

121. Nishikawa, R.M. and I.L. Chicago Univ. Cancers Missed on Mammography.2002;Available from: http://handle.dtic.mil/100.2/ADA411231

122. Jung, H., Is there a real risk of radiation-induced breast cancer for postmenopausal women? Radiation and environmental biophysics, 2001. 40(2): p. 169-74.

123. Wang, S.S., Researchers Create Better Ways to Spot Cancer Cells, in The Wall Street Journal 2011. p. 2.

124. Colborn,T.,D.Dumanoski,and J.P. Myers, Our stolen future:are we threatening our fertility, intelligence, and survival?:A scientific detective story 1996, New York: Duton.

125. Kaklamani, V., A genetic signature can predict prognosis and response to therapy in breast cancer: Oncotype DX. Expert-review-of-molecular diagnostics, 2006. 6(6): p. 803-9.

126. Retèl,V.P., et al.,Cost effectiveness of the 70 gene signture versus St. Gallen guidelines and Adjuvant Online for early breast cancer. European journal of cancer (Oxford, England : May, 2010), 2009. 46(8): p. 1382-91.

127. Ratner, E., et al., A KRAS-variant in ovarian cancer acts as a genetic marker of cancer risk. Cancer research, 2010. 70(16): p. 6509-15.

128. Chalothorn, L.A., et al., Hypodontia as a risk marker for epithelial ovarian cancer: A case controlled study. J Am Dent Assoc, 2008. 139(2): p. 163-169.

129. Elmore JG, B.M., Moceri VM, Polk S, Arena PJ, Fletcher SW., Ten year risk of false positive screening mammograms and clinical breast examinations. New England Journal of Medicine, 1998 Apr 16;. 338(16):1089-96

130. Laino, C. Blood Test for Cancer? 2006 [cited December 5,-2011];Available from: www.webmd.com/cancer/news/20060913/blood-test-for-cancer.

131. Lang, D.L.H., New Test Measures DNA Methylation Levels to Predict Colon Cancer Gastroenterology Gastroenterology, 2010.

Index

B

M

S

CPSIA information can be obtained at www.ICGtesting.com
Printed in the USA
LVOW101512270712

291876LV00005B/163/P